Epidurals for Childbirth

A Guide for All Delivery-Suite Staff
Second edition

Extensively revised and updated, the second edition of *Epidurals for Childbirth* offers a unique guide to the use of epidurals in obstetrics. Care has been taken to incorporate all recent changes to techniques and management in obstetric anaesthesia. The book presents clear, practical information and advice for all those involved in caring for women throughout pregnancy and labour. It is fully comprehensive, covering all medical aspects of epidurals, including anatomy, physiology and pharmacology. Concise explanations of practical procedures are provided along with potential problems and complications and how to handle them. Also included is a chapter on how to talk confidently to patients without using medical jargon. This book provides a valuable guide for all delivery-suite staff, including obstetricians, midwives, operating department practitioners and anaesthetists.

Anne May is Consultant Anaesthetist at Leicester Royal Infirmary and an Honorary Senior Lecturer at the University of Leicester.

Ralph Leighton is a Specialist Registrar in the Department of Anaesthesia, Critical Care and Pain Medicine at Leicester Royal Infirmary.

Epidurals for Childbirth

A Guide for All Delivery-Suite Staff

Second edition

ANNE MAY

RALPH LEIGHTON

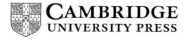

CAMBRIDGE
UNIVERSITY PRESS

CAMBRIDGE UNIVERSITY PRESS
Cambridge, New York, Melbourne, Madrid, Cape Town, Singapore, São Paulo

Cambridge University Press
The Edinburgh Building, Cambridge CB2 8RU, UK

Published in the United States of America by Cambridge University Press, New York

www.cambridge.org
Information on this title: www.cambridge.org/9780521704618

First published 2007

Printed in the United Kingdom at the University Press, Cambridge

A catalogue record for this publication is available from the British Library

ISBN 978-0-521-70461-8 paperback

Contents

Foreword

For trainee anaesthetists starting out in the wild, rugged territory of a labour ward, there can be nothing more reassuring than the presence of a calm, wise and experienced senior to show them the way and explain how and why things are done, or not done.

Those lucky enough to have worked with Anne May in their early years will know how well she has fitted this role, whilst for the rest of us 'of a certain age', there was the first edition of her book *Epidurals for Childbirth*, published in 1994, for comfort.

Small, friendly and refreshingly free of waffle, rather like its author, this book guided many a worried junior through tasks both routine and complex that lay in wait in the obstetric unit.

Now, after a long gap, Dr May together with her colleague Dr Leighton has revised and updated every aspect of the original to provide us with a new commonsensical and practical guide not only to epidurals, but to combined spinal epidurals and even general anaesthesia, explaining the day-to-day nuances that can mean the difference between success and failure, as well as preparing us for the exceptional cases. The book also covers what can go wrong, and what to do about it, though reading the first parts will make much of the later sections redundant. Non-anaesthetists can also benefit from the same sensible advice and explanations. Those who remember the original 'little green book' with fondness can once again refer to it (although it is no longer a 'little green book') while a new generation can discover its delights for the first time.

Steve Yentis
London

Acknowledgements

Our thanks go to both Donald and Emily for their support and understanding. We would like to thank Mr Paul Bosio an Dr Paul Sharpe for their assistance in the preparation of this book. We would also like to thank Dr Aung Gyi for his meticulous illustrations.

Pregnant women, their friends and their relatives may seek information about epidural analgesia from a variety of sources and this may lead to an incomplete and distorted view of pain relief in labour and in particular epidural analgesia. It is important that health care professionals are able to give sound answers to the many questions that they may be asked. Women need to be given accurate information in order to make an informed choice for their care during labour and delivery. It is to be recommended that a woman is well educated in the antenatal period so that she is able to give informed consent to an anaesthetic intervention even when she is in pain and distressed or has had opioid analgesia.

Why should the information be given?

The main reasons for giving information are to ensure that each woman is able to make informed choices about her labour and delivery and that she is able to give informed consent to an epidural if that is required. Normally verbal consent is obtained for epidural analgesia though it is much debated whether written consent is required. The medical notes should record the facts of the discussion and what information about risks and benefits was part of that conversation.

The best prelude to informed verbal consent is that the woman is knowledgeable about epidural analgesia before she arrives on the labour ward. The information must be understandable and take into account the language, intelligence and level of education of the woman. When epidural analgesia is discussed, all options of pain relief, with the risks and benefits of each should also be included. It is essential that this is a two-way process and that the woman is able to voice her concerns and have her questions answered. If the consultation was difficult because the woman was very distressed with pain then this should be recorded.

The main problems that relate to consent for epidural analgesia are that a large number of women may not intend to have an epidural and therefore do not feel it necessary to gain information about epidurals in the antenatal period. The problems arise when these women then cry out for an epidural when they are in pain and have had entonox and pethidine administered to them. It is exceedingly difficult to have a sensible discussion about pain relief and the risks and benefits of epidural analgesia in this situation though it could be said that consent in this case is implied as the woman needs to position herself for the procedure and to lie still. This situation is compounded if the woman does not speak English and though tempting to use the partner this is no substitute for a professional interpreter.

Birth plans or advance directives also cause problems and it could be argued that as the directive was written before the woman was aware how painful the labour would be, she should be able to change her mind in labour. A degree of common sense is needed in these situations. If the woman is almost fully dilated and is progressing well in a normal labour it is possibly wise to support her without an epidural, but if the labour is progressing abnormally and slowly then an epidural is possibly good practice to help the woman be in control.

The public has access to many sources of information and these include the internet, books, leaflets and magazines. Though a significant number are able to access good information easily there are still a significant number of women who are ill informed or denied access to information and the report of the Confidential Enquiry into Maternal Deaths highlights the problems of these disadvantaged women and in particular the problems of language and culture. Health care professionals must ensure that good lines of communication are in place at all levels of consultation throughout the antenatal period. Advice should be consistent and anaesthetists have a responsibility to ensure that our colleagues are well educated and know what information is recommended for the women.

Midwives have a responsibility to ensure that women with particular anxieties about epidural analgesia or medical problems have an anaesthetic consultation. Appropriate consultation can take place to discuss for example obesity, previous back surgery, cardiac disease, previous anaesthetic experience or particular fears. This consultation will allow a plan for analgesia and anaesthesia for labour and delivery to be set out and in the event of anaesthetic intervention being necessary the consent issue should be much easier.

How and when should the information be given?

Information should be readily available throughout the antenatal period using verbal, written and video material. The most important aspect is that all the health care professionals give accurate and consistent advice and are available to discuss questions about pain relief and in particular epidural analgesia. Midwives have a key role in helping women make informed choices about their place of delivery and decisions about the mode of delivery and pain relief.

The ideal time and place for talks and discussions about epidural analgesia is in the antenatal period and especially during parentcraft meetings when all aspects of pain relief in labour are covered. This type of group teaching is the most important way of reaching the majority of pregnant women, although at times it can be difficult to pitch information at a level that will be understood by all. For this reason the presence of an obstetric anaesthetist at selected parentcraft meetings allows questions to be asked and promotes discussion and better understanding of the issues.

Leaflets and videos provide an important source of additional information about epidural analgesia and they are usually on display at antenatal clinics and parentcraft meetings.

The Obstetric Anaesthetists Association (OAA) has worked hard to achieve these objectives in their pain relief booklet *Pain Relief in Labour* that has now sold over 250 000 copies and is available on the OAA website in over 17 languages. It is of great credit to the OAA that this booklet has been scored highly by the Centre for Health Information Quality. With the permission of the OAA the booklet is reproduced in Appendix C as an ideal for written information.

Although most pregnant women should have received all the information they need about epidural analgesia from parentcraft classes, there will be some women who ask specific questions arising from their personal circumstances at routine antenatal visits or during antenatal hospital admission. Medical and nursing staff should be able to answer such questions, and an obstetric anaesthetist should be available for consultation when the need arises. Planned analgesia should be the aim for women who have particular anxieties or medical problems.

By the time a pregnant woman reaches the delivery suite it is to her advantage that she already has a background of information about epidural analgesia, as this will allow an informed rational decision to be made early in labour should she request an epidural or should an epidural be recommended by a member of the delivery-suite team.

When this is not the case it can be difficult to explain the procedure of an epidural and the reasons why it is recommended to a distressed labouring woman. Explanations that can be given calmly and in full to a woman 'in control' may need to be modified or even directed to the partner of a woman who is 'out of control'.

The aim of informing all pregnant women about epidural analgesia in the antenatal period is that they arrive on the labour ward fully aware of what degree of pain relief an epidural can offer and how it will affect them and their labour. In many instances this information may lead to a planned epidural.

Information about the anaesthesia required for Caesarean section should also be available for all women in the antenatal period and is essential for those women who are to have a planned Caesarean delivery. This is recommended by the National Institute for Health and Clinical Excellence (NICE) in Clinical Guideline 13 – Caesarean section. The OAA has produced an information document, which is available on their website.

What information should be given?

Information should be made available to allow the pregnant woman and her partner to make informed choices about her labour and delivery. It is helpful to divide this information into four areas:

Anaesthetic service
Anaesthetist
Pain relief in labour
Anaesthesia.

Anaesthetic service

To make an informed choice about the place of delivery the woman should know what anaesthetic service is available. Some maternity units only have a limited obstetric anaesthetic service and may only run an on demand epidural service between certain hours. Others will have a dedicated obstetric anaesthetic consultant during those hours and outside those a dedicated resident anaesthetist for the delivery suite. To help make an informed choice, the woman may wish to ask the following questions: the epidural rate, Caesarean section rate, how long she can expect to wait to have an epidural sited, what the accidental dural puncture rate is, whether the women are followed up in the immediate postnatal period, and also whether there is the facility for postnatal follow-up at a later date for problems. Many obstetric anaesthetic services include the availability of an antenatal consultation with a consultant anaesthetist and these consultations are especially useful when the mother has particular anxieties or inter-current medical problems.

Anaesthetist

The general public is often unsure about the role of an anaesthetist within the maternity service and the following information may be useful. This information has been produced in a leaflet and it has been used on occasions where obstetric anaesthetists have run an open forum with the public.

Your anaesthetist in childbirth

An anaesthetist is part of the team that cares for you in pregnancy and child-birth. Your anaesthetist has a wide range of skills to help you when you have your baby and though everyone knows that anaesthetists give anaesthetics many people are unaware of the full role of the obstetric anaesthetist.

Most maternity units provide an epidural service. Ideally this is provided 24 hours a day, 365 days a year and run by obstetric anaesthetic consultants. A team of anaesthetists are available to administer epidural analgesia to women in labour. Also the anaesthetic team will be there to look after you if you need a Caesarean section and will encourage you to have a regional anaesthetic so that you can be awake for the delivery of your baby. A Caesarean delivery can therefore be a pleasurable birth experience with your partner present to support you and witness the birth.

Anaesthetists are highly trained in resuscitation and intensive care so if you are unfortunate enough to develop a serious complication of pregnancy then the obstetric anaesthetist is available to care for you. If you suffer from a medical condition an obstetric anaesthetist is often involved in planning your labour and delivery with the obstetric and midwifery staff and you may be asked to meet the anaesthetist in the antenatal period. Usually this is to advise on analgesia as we have a broad range of techniques to provide help with the pain of labour or the choice of anaesthesia if your delivery is to be by Caesarean section.

Pain relief in labour

Information about pain relief in labour should not focus on pain but rather the management of labour with dignity and control. It must be recognized that every labour is different and not all women want the same experience. Some women want to experience pain though others wish to have a pain-free labour and our role is to help women make the right choice. It is also vitally important that the woman remains flexible in her outlook to avoid disappointment and that those women who have a medical reason for epidural analgesia are appropriately managed. The OAA has made information to mothers a priority and the *Pain Relief in Labour* leaflet is appended at the end of this book (see Appendix C). Information should be available about all methods of pain relief and include an unbiased discussion of the risks and benefits of each technique. It is important that the language is appropriate for the level of understanding and education of the woman and translations and interpreters are widely available.

Frequently asked questions

Does it work?

Yes, it is the best pain relief available. It may take a little time to produce complete pain relief (i.e. a perfect block) in all women. The aim is a pain-free labour. Failure to achieve this may be due to the epidural's being put in place too late, in which case the anaesthetic effect has insufficient time to work before delivery. Recent developments have shown that epidural analgesia can be used to modify pain and allow the woman to remain ambulant.

How does it work?

Epidural analgesia works by blocking the transmission of impulses in the nerves that carry the sensation of pain from the uterus and birth canal to the brain. The local anaesthetic is placed around the nerves in the epidural space – a space outside the spinal cord.

Is it safe?

Yes, but like all procedures it carries a small risk of complications that can be explained to you. (This question may first be approached by emphasizing the general safety of the obstetric unit with particular reference to staff available – ideally 24-hour resident-designated cover.)

Specific questions about safety are usually related to minor complications such as a headache or residual areas of numbness, or to the possibility of serious complications such as paralysis, coma or even death. (These topics are dealt with later.)

Minor complications

Headache: A headache can be caused by accidental puncture of the dura – the membrane surrounding the spinal cord – this is not life-threatening and can be regarded as a nuisance. If this complication occurs, you should be told immediately and a full explanation of the best way to treat it will be given.

There is a risk of dural puncture associated with epidural analgesia and the overall incidence is around 0.5–1.0%. (Only half of these will go on to develop a headache if treated appropriately, that is the overall incidence of dural-puncture headache is about 0.25–0.50%.)

Areas of numbness: Areas of numbness are most commonly due to a circumstance of the birth, for example a forceps delivery or the pressure on your legs from the apparatus that supports them during delivery rather than the epidural itself. You should report any such areas of numbness to the anaesthetist or midwife. However, occasionally areas of numbness in the legs can remain for some time after the epidural – anything from a day to several weeks. They resolve in due course.

Serious complications

Serious complications from an epidural are extremely rare. Specific worries about the risk of serious complications such as paralysis, coma or even death resulting from an epidural are occasionally voiced. Quantification of these risks may be helpful – one study suggests 1 in 100 000 epidurals. The general safety of the unit and the immediate availability of an anaesthetist can again be emphasized.

Will it hurt?

Inserting an epidural is sometimes uncomfortable but not usually painful. However, you will feel some sensations and these can be fully explained to you by describing the various stages of the procedure.

Position
You will either be curled up on your side or bent forward in the sitting position. You must remain still as the epidural space is small and the procedure is delicate.

Timing
It is easier to insert the epidural before you are in too much pain, but it is never too late to ask for an epidural; although in some circumstances an epidural may not be appropriate.

Preparation
Your back is cleaned and draped and a small amount of local anaesthetic is injected into the skin overlying the area where the epidural will be inserted, that is between the bony bumps (spinous processes) at about waist level. This may sting a little but it makes the rest of the procedure more comfortable.

Insertion of the epidural needle
The needle used to detect the epidural space will be inserted between the spinous processes. The only sensation that you will feel here is pressure on your back. Once the epidural space is found, the catheter – a fine polythene tube – is inserted through the needle; this may produce a strange sensation or a feeling of 'pins and needles'. The needle is removed and the catheter is left in place and firmly attached to your skin with sticky tape.

Administering the epidural anaesthetic
First, a test dose of anaesthetic is injected through the catheter to ensure that you do not react adversely to it. Once this is established the next dose is given, which may take up to 20 minutes to have its full effect. When the anaesthetic has taken full effect you should be pain free, but you will still be aware of your contractions. You should also be aware of the presence of the baby's head during delivery.

Top-up doses of anaesthetic
Top-up doses are usually necessary every 30–60 minutes. Each dose is given through the catheter by the midwife or anaesthetist and the administration

of each dose is painless. A stronger top-up of an epidural already in place can give sufficient anaesthesia for a forceps delivery or a Caesarean section if either becomes necessary during your labour.

Will it damage or affect my baby?

No, only a minute amount of the local anaesthetic may reach your baby via your blood stream. The effect of this is practically zero and is very much less than the effect of pethidine or other pain-killing drugs that you may be given for a painful labour without an epidural. Epidural analgesia will not affect your ability to breast feed and may enhance it.

Will I be able to push?

Yes, but your second stage of labour will be managed differently if an epidural is in place. Without an epidural, pushing usually begins as soon as the cervix is fully dilated, that is at the beginning of the second stage of labour. With an epidural in place, you may not experience the urge to push at this stage. Instead, the baby's head will naturally continue its passage through the birth canal aided by the normal contractions of your womb. You should feel the urge to push when the baby's head is near delivery, and you will then be encouraged to push actively to enjoy a normal childbirth.

Will I need an instrumental delivery if I have an epidural?

Not necessarily. However, an epidural may have been recommended to you in the first place because there are circumstances connected with the birth of your baby that may in themselves make a forceps delivery more likely.

Will it damage my back?

No, minor back problems are common after childbirth with or without an epidural. Epidurals are themselves used to treat many chronic back conditions.

If you happen to suffer from any back complaint, for example a previous operation on your spine, a slipped disc (disc prolapse), or a twisted or bent spine (scoliosis), you should tell the anaesthetist or midwife. Back problems such as these can make the giving of an epidural technically more difficult, but they are not a contraindication.

Will I be able to move my legs?

While the epidural is working, you may experience temporary difficulty in moving your legs. The dose of local anaesthetic can be adjusted to minimize this effect, and recent developments may allow you to walk about with the epidural in place.

Do I really need an epidural?

You may choose to have an epidural simply to enjoy a pain-free labour. However, an epidural may be recommended to you, by a doctor or midwife, if you have or develop a particular problem in pregnancy or during childbirth. If this is the case the need for an epidural will be explained to you.

What if it is suggested that I have an epidural?

The obstetricians, midwives and anaesthetists looking after you may suggest that an epidural would be helpful for a variety of good reasons and they will explain these fully to you. If you require a Caesarean section epidurals are encouraged in preference to general anaesthesia enabling you to see your baby at the moment of birth and allowing you to participate in the birth.

Anaesthesia

Most women do not believe that they will need an anaesthetic during childbirth. However with a Caesarean section rate of around 20% and rising, a significant number of women will have an anaesthetic either for a Caesarean section or for other medical reasons. All women should know the risks and benefits of general and regional anaesthesia and know what percentage of women are delivered under regional anaesthesia in the unit they are booked in. Information leaflets should be available in all units. The OAA has recently produced a leaflet on Caesarean section called *Caesarean section: your choice of anaesthesia* (which is reproduced in Appendix D) and also a video and DVD.

Regional anaesthesia can be achieved by an epidural top-up, a spinal or combined spinal epidural. These techniques are described in Chapter 12. Whichever technique is used the woman should be informed of the risks of headache, failure, pruritis, nausea and vomiting, and hypotension. She should understand that during the procedure she will feel a degree of pushing and pulling and if at any stage she is uncomfortable then the anaesthetist will be with her to support her and administer medication to her. The woman should also be informed about the administration of syntocinon to help the placenta separate and the uterus contract, the need for prophylactic antibiotics, thromboprophylaxis and the provision of post-operative pain relief.

Even in the emergency situation the delivery of the baby by Caesarean section with regional anaesthesia should be a pleasurable birth experience, with the woman and her partner able to see the delivery of their baby and to have close contact with the baby as soon as possible after delivery.

Despite all our efforts, however, some women go into labour with prejudiced opinions about epidurals and regional anaesthesia based on information, which is often biased and anecdotal, gleaned from the popular press and women's magazines, or the internet. When the aim of comprehensive, balanced information available to all is achieved, women will at last have a full choice of pain relief in labour and be well informed about regional anaesthesia if they need a Caesarean section.

The OAA (www.oaa-anaes.ac.uk) has made providing information to mothers a priority and continues to help women make informed choices about their management of analgesia and anaesthesia in childbirth.

2 Anatomy of the epidural space

Epidural analgesia is a procedure whereby local anaesthetic solution is placed around the nerves as they cross the epidural space from the uterus and birth canal to the spinal cord in order to relieve the pain of labour and childbirth. The segmental nerves involved are from T12 to L1–2 for analgesia in the first stage of labour and from S2 to S4 for analgesia in the second stage of labour. A full description of the nerve supply to the uterus and birth canal is given in Chapter 7.

A working knowledge of the anatomy of the epidural space and the structures around it is essential for those who perform epidurals and for those who are involved in the care of women with an epidural in place. For the anaesthetist wishing to learn the technique of epidural analgesia a clear three-dimensional knowledge of the structures through which the epidural needle must pass before reaching the epidural space will be enormously helpful.

This chapter sets out to achieve this by describing the anatomy step by step in the following order:

Skeleton of the lumbar spine
Ligaments through which the epidural needle passes
Epidural space
Spinal cord and its coverings.

Skeleton of the lumbar spine

In order to place local anaesthetic around the nerves in the epidural space it is necessary to know exactly the position of these nerves in relation to the bony landmarks of the spine. The main requirement of an epidural is pain relief for the first stage of labour, and for this the lumbar route is the most logical. The spaces most commonly used to approach the epidural space are L2–3 and L3–4 for two reasons: the spinal cord ends at around L1 in adults; and the lumbar lordosis is greatest at L5–S1. The spinal cord and epidural space are well protected by the vertebral column and its attached ligaments. The bony landmarks shown in Fig. 2.1 are helpful for finding the interspaces between the L2, L3 and L4 spinous processes.

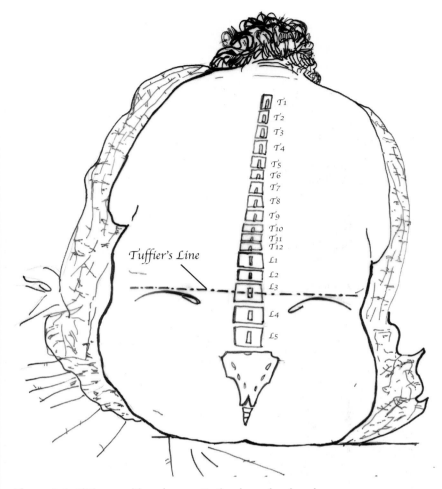

T1
T2
T3
T4
T5
T6
T7
T8
T9
T10
T11
T12
L1
L2
L3
L4
L5

Tuffier's Line

Figure 2.1 Sitting position demonstrating bony landmarks

When locating the lumbar spinous processes, a mental picture of the anatomy of the lumbar vertebrae is an advantage see Fig. 2.2. There are five lumbar vertebrae, and as their function is weight bearing they are strong structures.

The body of each lumbar vertebra is in the shape of a truncated wedge with the thick end anterior to the thin end, thus producing the normal lumbar lordosis. This is most pronounced at L5–S1 as a result of which the approach to the epidural space becomes more awkward at this level.

The intervertebral discs (the 'shock absorbers' of the spinal column) are also wedge shaped, contributing to the lumbar lordosis, and they are made up of two parts: a peripheral fibrous portion (annulus fibrosus) and a central gelatinous portion (nucleus pulposus).

The lumbar vertebrae and intervertebral discs are shown in Fig. 2.3.

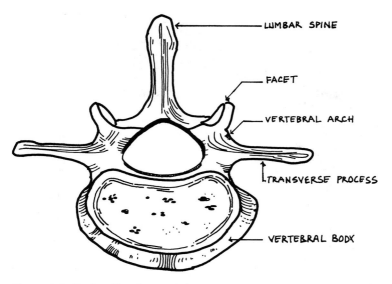

Figure 2.2 Body of lumbar vertebra

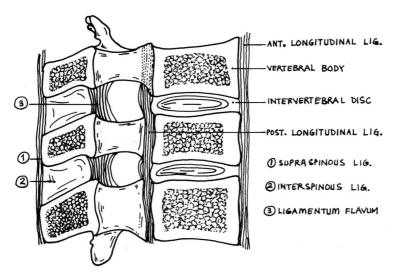

Figure 2.3 Lumbar vertebrae and intervertebral discs (ANT.: anterior; POST.: posterior; LIG.: ligament)

Ligaments of the vertebral column

The vertebral arch, its attachments and its related structures are very important in epidural analgesia. The ligaments of the vertebral column bind the vertebrae together and have an important function in maintaining the erect posture, thus sparing muscular effort.

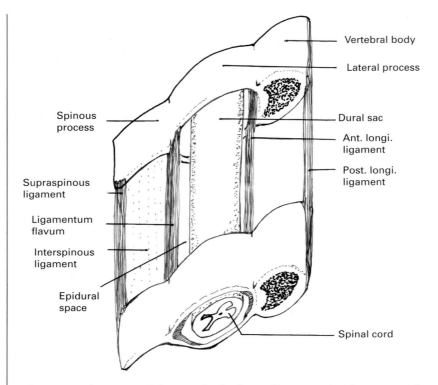

Figure 2.4 Ligaments of the vertebral column (Ant.: anterior; Post.: posterior; Longi.: longitudinal)

The ligaments supporting the vertebral column are as shown in Fig. 2.4.

Supraspinous ligament

The supraspinous ligament is a moderately tough taut band of fibres that spans the tips of the spinous processes from C7 to the sacrum. Its thickest and widest portion is in the lumbar region and it offers the first resistance to the epidural needle.

Interspinous ligament

The interspinous ligament is a low-density collection of fibres connecting and occupying the space between the spinous processes. It merges with the supraspinous ligament and the ligamentum flavum. The interspinous ligament offers less resistance to the epidural needle than the supraspinous ligament, but it does provide some support to the needle that is helpful to the anaesthetist as he or she advances the needle towards the ligamentum flavum. The interspinous ligament has less substance below L4. Therefore at this level it becomes technically more difficult to site an epidural owing to a reduction in the support offered by the ligament to the needle. This loss of support may amount to a sensation of false 'loss of resistance' (see below) as the needle pierces the supraspinous ligament.

Ligamentum flavum

The ligamentum flavum (the yellow ligament) is made up of elastic fibres that extend laterally from the bases of the spinous processes to blend with the joint capsules of the articular processes. It runs from the anterior inferior surface of the lamina above to the posterior superior surface of the lamina below. The distance between the skin and the ligamentum flavum averages 6 cm. This may be reduced to 3 cm in slim young women, but may be as great as 10 cm in obese women.

The ligament is 2–5 mm thick and its thickest part is in the lumbar region. There is thinning of the ligament which is a V-shaped structure at the mid-line to allow for the passage of blood vessels, but in practice this does not affect the 'loss of resistance' described below as the epidural needle is rarely, if ever, positioned exactly at the mid-line.

The ligamentum flavum provides the greatest resistance to the epidural needle. When the needle is in the ligamentum flavum it is normally held firmly in place and as the needle is advanced the resistance is overcome and a loss of resistance is felt as the epidural space is entered.

However, there is considerable variation in the 'feel' of the ligament between women. In general all ligaments are softened in pregnancy owing to the influence of progesterone, but the ligamentum flavum may be particularly soft in women suffering from pre-eclampsia or in the obese woman. The 'feel' in such cases can be compared with pushing a needle through butter. Conversely, it is a personal observation of the authors that in sportswomen the ligamentum flavum can be very firm or even tough to the extent that a considerable amount of effort is required to pass the epidural needle through it.

Anterior and posterior ligaments

The anterior and posterior longitudinal ligaments are bound to the anterior and posterior surfaces respectively of the vertebral bodies and run from C2 to the sacrum. They are not traversed by the epidural needle.

Table 2.1 Boundaries of the epidural space

Above	the foramen magnum. Here the periosteal and the meningeal layers of the cerebral dura fuse together. Therefore local anaesthetic solution that has been placed in the epidural space will not extend higher than the foramen magnum.
Below	the sacrococcygeal membrane.
In front	the posterior longitudinal ligament, to which the spinal dura is loosely attached by fibrous bands.
Behind	the ligamentum flavum and the vertebral laminae.
Laterally	the pedicles of the vertebra and the intervertebral foraminae.

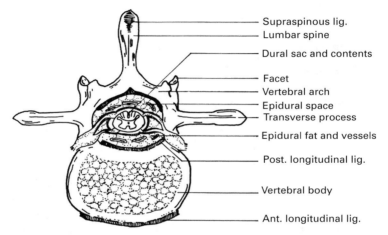

Supraspinous lig.
Lumbar spine

Dural sac and contents

Facet
Vertebral arch
Epidural space
Transverse process

Epidural fat and vessels

Post. longitudinal lig.

Vertebral body

Ant. longitudinal lig.

Figure 2.5 The epidural space (ANT.: anterior; POST.: posterior; LIG.: ligament)

Epidural space

The epidural space is the column formed between the periosteal lining of the vertebral canal and the spinal dura mater. It contains spinal nerve roots, lymphatic ducts, blood vessels and a variable amount of fat, see Fig. 2.5.

Boundaries of the epidural space

These are shown in Table 2.1.

The epidural space can therefore be described as a tube. The epidural space is oval in the lumbar region becoming triangular in the lower lumbar region. At the centre of this tube is a second tube, which is formed by the meninges and contains the spinal cord and the cerebrospinal fluid that bathes it. However, the epidural space is a leaky tube as it is crossed by

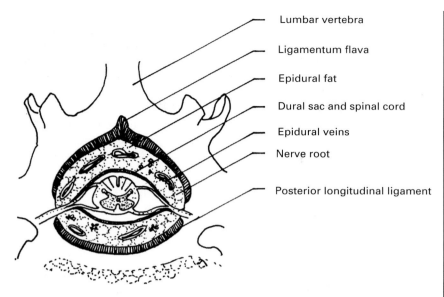

Lumbar vertebra

Ligamentum flava

Epidural fat

Dural sac and spinal cord

Epidural veins

Nerve root

Posterior longitudinal ligament

Figure 2.6 Contents of the epidural space

31 spinal nerves that, together with their coverings of dura mater, pass through the intervertebral foraminae to the paravertebral space.

In elderly people the tube becomes less leaky, but in the young pregnant woman there will be free interconnection between the epidural space and the paravertebral space, so that local anaesthetic can travel freely from the epidural space to the paravertebral space. This may have the effect of dispersing the anaesthetic solution, thus producing an ineffective block.

The portion of dura mater that is attached to the posterior longitudinal ligament (see Fig. 2.5) may have centrally placed folds. This anatomical variation may explain the problem of a complete unilateral block, but the evidence for this is not conclusive.

Contents of the lumbar epidural space

The contents of the lumbar epidural space are shown in Fig. 2.6.

Fatty tissue

The amount of fatty tissue in the epidural space is proportional to the adiposity of the woman. The presence of fat is relevant to epidural analgesia as fatty tissue will take up lipid-soluble drugs such as local anaesthetics. This 'mopping up' of local anaesthetic solution will leave less available to act on the nerve roots.

Epidural veins

The epidural veins form the venous plexus of the vertebral canal. They lie mainly in the antero-lateral part of the epidural space and run vertically, draining into the azygos system. The azygos system can become an important route of venous return for the lower part of the body, particularly when the inferior vena cava may be compressed as in pregnancy. As the azygos veins drain into the superior vena cava and thence directly to the heart, it is important to note that local anaesthetic solution injected inadvertently into an epidural vein could rapidly reach the heart with potentially dangerous effects (these are fully described in Chapter 10). In such an event, the greater the obstruction to the inferior vena cava, the greater would be the concentration of local anaesthetic that would reach the heart.

As performing an epidural is essentially a blind procedure there is no certain way of avoiding accidental perforation or cannulation of an engorged epidural vein.

The resulting complications are as follows:

1. Accidental intravenous injection of local anaesthetic solution (as discussed above).
2. Bleeding into the epidural space. The presence of blood in the epidural space can prevent the even spread of local anaesthetic solution even after successful epidural cannulation. If the bleeding is uncontrolled, a haematoma may develop resulting in a build-up of pressure in the epidural space sufficient to cause spinal cord or nerve root compression.

The management of these complications is fully described in Chapter 10.

Epidural arteries

The epidural arteries in the lumbar region of the epidural space are branches of the ilio-lumbar arteries. They lie in the lateral part of the epidural space and therefore are outside the path of an advancing epidural needle.

Spinal nerves

The spinal nerves from segments T10–S5 pass through the epidural space and are readily accessible via the lumbar epidural route.

Spinal cord and its coverings

The spinal cord runs within the epidural space contained by the protective meninges and ends at level L1 or L2 in the conus medullaris. Below this it becomes a leash of lumbar and sacral nerve roots (the cauda equina) and filum terminale. The cord is bathed in a fluid (the cerebrospinal fluid) that is contained within the meninges.

The meninges are comprised of three layers, the outmost dura mater, the arachnoid mater and the innermost pia mater, which is adherent to the spinal cord.

The dura mater is a dense inelastic membrane, which for practical purposes can be divided into two entities: (i) the cerebral dura mater; (ii) the spinal dura mater. The cerebral dura mater comprises two layers: the outer (periosteal) layer and the inner (meningeal) layer, which invests the brain. These two layers are in close apposition except where the venous sinuses that supply the brain lie between them. The outer layer of the cerebral dura is itself closely applied to the periosteum of the cranium but it becomes firmly adherent to the periosteum at the foramen magnum.

The spinal dura mater is a continuation of the meningeal layer of the cerebral dura mater and it forms a loose tube around the spinal cord. The periosteal layer of the cerebral dura ceases at the foramen magnum below which it becomes the periosteal lining of the vertebral canal. The dural tube continues below the lower end of the spinal cord as far as S2 and below this level there is no fluid. At S2 the dura becomes part of the filum terminale externa, which blends with the periosteum on the back of the coccyx.

The distance between the posterior and anterior walls of the dura as approached by the epidural needle at approximately the mid-line (at level L2 to L5) is between 4–8 mm.

The dura mater and the underlying arachnoid mater can be separated to form the subdural space. If local anaesthetic solution were to be injected into this space it would spread extensively, producing a widespread 'sub-dural' nerve blockade.

Blood supply of the spinal cord

The anterior spinal artery runs in the anterior median fissure of the cord and supplies the anterior two thirds of the cord. Ischaemia of this part of the spinal cord will cause weakness in the lower body and a patchy sensory loss.

Posterior spinal arteries descend along each side of the cord anterior and posterior to the dorsal nerve roots.

Radicular branches come from local arteries and feed into the spinal arteries.

Further comments on anatomy

Our understanding of the anatomy of the epidural space and spinal cord has been enhanced by epiduroscopy and especially by magnetic resonance imaging (MRI).

It is hoped that the description of the anatomy of the epidural space will emphasize that a working knowledge of the anatomy is essential before the placement of an epidural is carried out. This knowledge reinforces the fact that placing an epidural catheter and local anaesthetic solution in the epidural space is not the simple procedure that it may appear to be.

Despite the close proximity of all the anatomical structures, the leaky nature of the epidural tube and the possible anatomical variations that may be encountered, epidural analgesia is a surprisingly safe and effective procedure. A clear understanding of the anatomy will help the anaesthetist to solve problems that may occur during positioning the woman, inserting the epidural and topping up the epidural. Such problems are explained in detail in Chapters 3, 7 and 10.

3 Performing an epidural

Introduction

Epidural analgesia is the best analgesia available for childbirth, Therefore, the prime indication for epidural analgesia is the treatment of pain. We know that 75% of first-time mothers have enough pain for them to request pain relief and in some the pain is so severe that they need epidural analgesia early in labour. There is evidence to suggest that severe labour pain is a marker for an abnormal labour although there is continuing debate about the cause and effect of epidural analgesia on the mode of delivery of the baby. Previous concerns have largely been dispelled (see Chapter 7). Though the majority of requests for epidural analgesia arise in labour there are many women who have known medical or obstetric problems where epidural analgesia is indicated for their delivery (see Chapters 8 and 9)

The obstetric indications for epidural analgesia can be discussed in three groups that relate to the time the need is recognized and these are the antenatal period, intrapartum and postpartum.

Antenatal:

- breech presentation
- twin pregnancy
- intrauterine growth retardation
- pregnancy induced hypertension (including pre-eclampsia)
- intrauterine death or termination of an abnormal fetus
- inter-current medical problems in the mother
- previous Caesarean section.

Intrapartum:

- pain
- maternal request
- induction of labour
- slow progress in labour
- augmentation of labour with syntocinon
- the need for fetal blood sampling
- occipito posterior position and other malpresentations

- instrumental delivery
- pre-term delivery (labour).

Postpartum

- suturing
- manual removal of retained placenta.

Contraindications to epidural analgesia

1. Patient refusal
2. Sepsis at the site where the epidural would be placed
3. Untreated systemic sepsis
4. Significant bleeding disorders.

Performing an epidural

All staff working in a delivery suite should have a basic knowledge of the equipment and techniques used for performing an epidural. It is essential that the delivery-suite team have a clear understanding of the procedure so that they are able to offer positive support to the labouring woman and to the anaesthetist. Performing an epidural will be discussed under the following headings.

- Equipment for epidural analgesia
- Preparation for epidural analgesia
- Steps involved in performing an epidural
- Difficulties encountered during placing an epidural.

Equipment for epidural analgesia

- intravenous (IV) cannula, giving set and fluid
- gown, gloves, mask and hat
- skin antiseptic
- sterile drapes
- syringe and needles for local anaesthetic infiltration
- local anaesthetic and saline solutions
- epidural needle
- epidural catheter
- filter (0.2 μm)
- loss of resistance device
- scalpel blade (optional)
- adhesive dressing.

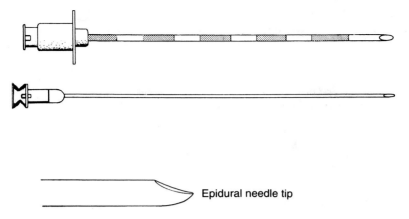

Epidural needle tip

Figure 3.1 Tuohy needle and stilette

The only specialized items of equipment in the above list are the epidural needle, the epidural catheter, the filter and the loss of resistance device. These are described in detail below.

The epidural needle

An epidural needle is blunt and has an angled end to facilitate the insertion of a catheter through its lumen. The most popular needle is the Tuohy needle. The Tuohy needle is 18, 17 or 16 gauge and the most frequently used size in the UK is 16 gauge. The needle usually has centimetre markings along its 8 cm length with 11 cm needles available for use in larger women. A removable stilette slots down the centre of the needle, and the hub is produced with or without wings or optionally attachable wings. The distal portion of the needle that is first inserted into the woman is blunt and curved as illustrated in Fig. 3.1. Bluntness is essential for the detection of the ligamentum flavum during insertion. A sharp needle would cut through the ligament without the operator sensing the resistance that indicates that the ligament has been reached.

The catheter

The catheter is designed to thread through the positioned epidural needle into the epidural space. It is usually made of flexible polyvinyl plastic and is specially manufactured to minimize the possibility of causing trauma within the epidural space. The portion that is inserted into the epidural space should not be sharp and should thread easily through and out of the needle. Small holes are present at the end of the catheter to allow free flow of the local anaesthetic in the epidural space.

The filter

All solutions should first be filtered through a 0.2 μm filter to ensure that no bacteria or debris are introduced into the epidural space, in particular glass particles from glass ampoules.

Loss of resistance device

The most commonly used device for detecting loss of resistance on entering the epidural space is a minimal resistance syringe. Traditionally this was made of glass. There are several brands of disposable loss of resistance plastic syringes available on the market. Historically, various other methods and devices have been used to detect loss of resistance, for example the Macintosh balloon and the hanging drop technique.

Preparation for epidural analgesia

The anaesthetist and midwife, and on some occasions an operating department practitioner, are all involved in preparing the woman for an epidural. The midwife and/or obstetrician may have instigated the discussion about pain relief and the recommendation of an epidural. Ideally the woman should have been well informed in the antenatal period and have an understanding of what an epidural is, and what it entails including the risks and benefits of the procedure. The anaesthetist must ascertain what information the woman has had and be reassured that she consents to the procedure. The problems of providing information to women and the problems of consent in distressed labouring women are covered in Chapter 1. The anaesthetist will need to introduce himself to the woman and familiarize himself with the medical and obstetric history while obtaining consent to the epidural from the woman. Once the decision has been made for the epidural to be sited the following should be checked:

- blood pressure
- blood tests where relevant
- fetal well-being, from the history and cardiotocograph (CTG) or fetal blood samples
- that the woman is suitably dressed
- that the bladder has been emptied recently
- 16G intravenous cannula is sited
- suitable intravenous fluid is running, see Chapter 6.

The next event is to position the woman. The correct positioning of the woman is very important and may require the help of both the midwife and the partner. The woman can either be sitting or curled up on her side in the left lateral position. As far as the comfort of the woman is concerned there is little to choose between these two positions though obese woman may

Table 3.1 Comparison of sitting and lying positions

Sitting up	Lying (left lateral)
Advantages	
Mid-line easier to identify in obese women	Can be left unattended without risk of fainting
Obese patients may find this position more comfortable	No orthostatic hypotension
	Utero-placental blood flow not reduced (particular important in the stressed fetus)
Disadvantages	
Utero-placental blood flow decreased	May be more difficult to find the mid-line in obese patients
Orthostatic hypotension may occur	
Increased risk of orthostatic hypotension if entonox and pethidine have been administered	
Patient sitting on edge of bed may be too far away from a small anaesthetist for good manual dexterity	
Assistant (or partner) needed to support patient	

become dyspnoeic on their side. The advantages and disadvantages of both positions are summarized in Table 3.1.

In either position, the spine should be well flexed with the hips and shoulders aligned, and this can be facilitated by telling the woman to 'roll up like a hedgehog' or 'arch her back like an angry cat'. In the sitting position the woman's knees should be placed aside rather than underneath her 'bump', asking the woman to pretend to 'sit on the back pockets of her trousers' may be helpful. The woman is now ready. See Figs. 3.2–3.4.

Steps involved in performing an epidural

The assistant

The assistant should give support to the woman and the anaesthetist throughout the procedure. They should work with the anaesthetist and be aware of the stage of the procedure at all times while monitoring the uterine contractions. It is recommended that the fetal heart be monitored throughout the placement of the epidural though it is recognized that when external monitoring is used it may often be impracticable for some of the time.

The assistant should understand the importance of a sterile technique and be ready to assist the anaesthetist in opening sterile packs. The assistant

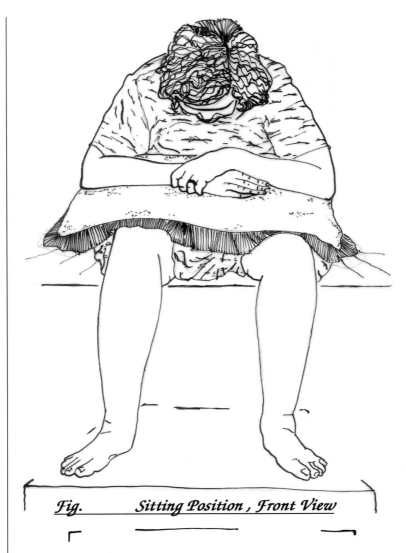

Figure 3.2 Bony landmarks with the patient in the sitting position –
anterior–posterior view

should ensure the woman's position is optimal. Once the epidural is sited
the assistant should then help in fixing the epidural catheter to the woman's
back, and to monitor the woman.

The anaesthetist
Performing an epidural is a sterile procedure. The anaesthetist should wear
a hat and mask, wash his hands thoroughly, and put on a gown and surgical

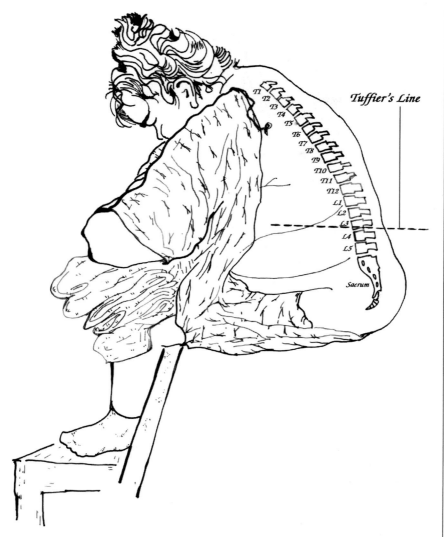

Figure 3.3 Bony landmarks with the patient in the sitting position – lateral view

gloves. Once the anaesthetist has checked the equipment, the woman, anaesthetist and assistant are now ready.

- Check the woman's position.
- Clean the woman's back, usually with chlorhexidine in alcohol. There is less likelihood of the chlorhexidine coming into contact with the epidural needle or catheter if the chlorhexidine is sprayed directly onto the woman's back by the assistant rather than being swabbed onto the

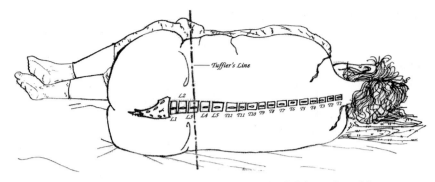

Figure 3.4 Bony landmarks with the patient in the left lateral position

woman from a galley pot on the epidural trolley. The solution should be allowed to dry. An 'ozone friendly' pump spray can be used rather than a pressurized aerosol.

- Check the bony landmarks.
- Cover the woman's back with sterile drapes.
- Choose the best suitable interspinous space L2–3, L3–4 or L4–5. Remember the position of the cord in relation to Tuffier's line.
- Raise a wheal of local anaesthetic (lignocaine 2%) then infiltrate the subcutaneous tissues with local anaesthetic taking care not to enter the epidural space.
- A small nick may be made in the infiltrated skin with a number 11 scalpel blade to avoid skin being taken into the epidural space with the epidural needle (optional).
- Gently advance a Tuohy needle through the skin nick. It is important to have a mental picture of the position of the end of the needle as it is inserted (see Chapter 2). The needle is advanced in the direction of the ligamentum flavum whose fibres it will either cut through when the bevel is at right angles to the spine or pushed apart when the bevel is in line with the spine. The needle will be firmly held in the ligamentum flavum (Fig. 3.5). It is a matter of individual choice whether the face of the bevel is advanced laterally to the mid-line or cephalad. In the former case the catheter will tend to thread laterally and in the latter it will tend to thread along the mid-line. Once the needle has entered the epidural space it should not be rotated as this is associated with an increased risk of puncturing the dura.
- The hands should be placed so that the needle is supported at all times allowing fine control of the advancement of the needle by the fingers.
- Remove the stilette from the needle before the ligamentum flavum is broached and place a syringe (filled with either saline or air) on the end of the needle. (The advantages and disadvantages of saline and air are compared in Table 3.2.)

Table 3.2 Comparison of saline and air

Saline	Air
Advantages	
May give a better end point for loss of resistance	If fluid appears during insertion it can be assumed to be CSF until proved otherwise
May push the dura away from the point of the needle thus reducing the chances of dural puncture	No filter is required
	No dilutional effects; the small amount of air used does not usually distort the tissues
	No possibility of confusion with other substances
Disadvantages	
May be confused with CSF	More difficult to define the point of loss of resistance with air than with saline
Must be filtered to avoid introduction of minute glass particles	
Dilutes the local anaesthetic which is put into the epidural space	
Another ampoule is opened, thus providing a possibility for user error	
Preservative-free saline must be used (NB alcohol may be present as a preservative)	

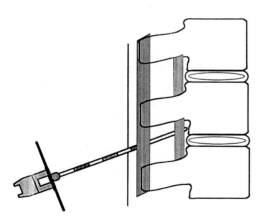

Figure 3.5 Needle in the ligamentum flavum

- Advance the needle slowly with simultaneous continuous or intermittent pressure on the syringe plunger. If saline is used the pressure should be continuous. Loss of resistance indicates that the epidural space has been entered. The tip of the needle is now in the epidural space.

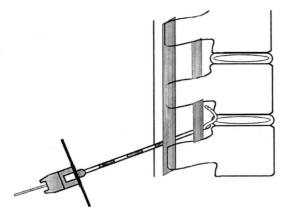

Figure 3.6 Illustration to show the successful threading of the catheter into the epidural space

- If fluid flows freely back from the epidural needle, then it is possible that the needle has travelled too far and punctured the dura (see below).
- Instruct the woman to remain still during catheter insertion and warn her that she may feel a sensation of 'pins and needles' in her back or legs.
- Remove the syringe and thread the catheter through the needle. The introducer may assist in the smooth threading of the catheter.
- The catheter should thread without force once through the end of the needle (Fig. 3.6). *It must not be withdrawn through the needle* as it may be damaged or sheared, leaving a piece of catheter in the woman. If there is acute pain or resistance to the catheter during threading *come out* (that is, remove epidural needle and catheter together) and *start again*. Take care to thread a generous length of catheter (at least 5 cm) beyond the distal end of the needle in the epidural space. It is best to err on the long side as the catheter can always be withdrawn a little after removal of the needle.
- Remove the needle, taking care not to remove or displace the catheter at the same time, and connect the end of the catheter to the filter. Adjust the length to 3–4 cm. This is important because if the catheter is too short it will tend to fall out, and if it is too long a unilateral block is more likely. If the woman is obese the catheter is more likely to displace and so 4–6 cm should be left in the epidural space.
- Attach the syringe and gently aspirate the catheter to check that no blood or cerebrospinal fluid (CSF) is withdrawn.
- Secure the catheter firmly to the woman's back.
- Give the test dose of local anaesthetic.

Test doses

The administration of a test dose of local anaesthetic prior to the full dose is a safety measure carried out by the majority of anaesthetists to check the correct placement of the epidural catheter. The response to the test dose should ideally indicate whether the catheter is in the epidural space or whether it has accidentally threaded into a blood vessel or through the dura into the CSF. Commonly used test doses are 2–3 ml bupivacaine 0.5%, 1.5–2 ml lignocaine 2%, or 5–10 mls of 0.1% bupivacaine with 2 μg of fentanyl per ml.

Response to correct placement of catheter

There should be no response to the test dose after 5 minutes.

Response to intrathecal placement of the catheter

- dramatic relief of pain (if in labour)
- drop in blood pressure
- some motor block.

Response to intravascular placement of catheter

If the catheter is accidentally placed in an epidural vein, a positive response to a test dose of local anaesthetic is often not convincing. The symptoms that suggest a positive response are a metallic test in the mouth and tinnitus. Circumoral pallor may also be observed.

Some centres (notably in the USA) use a very small dose (15 μg) of adrenaline 1:1000 alone or mixed with the local anaesthetic test dose to test for accidental intravascular catheterization. This is monitored by an electrocardiogram (ECG), and a rise in maternal heart rate of more than 25 beats/minute after one minute is significant. This method may not be practical as a distressed woman will have a rapidly varying pulse rate in response to pain.

Limitations of test doses

Test doses are not completely reliable, and so even with a negative response the full dose of epidural anaesthetic should be given slowly and cautiously with continued observation for signs of intrathecal or intravascular placement of the catheter.

Difficulties encountered during placing an epidural

The 'moving target'

A distressed or anxious woman causing a 'moving target' requires an authoritative approach from both the midwife/assistant and the anaesthetist.

Difficulty in finding the interspinous spaces

This is particularly likely in the obese or in the oedematous woman. Checking the position of the woman and repositioning if necessary may solve the

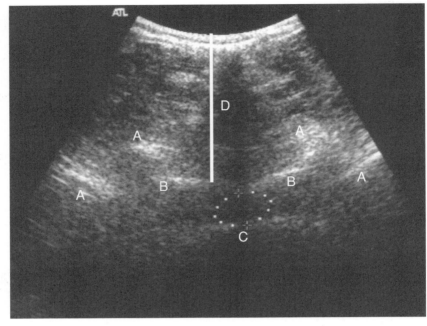

Legend

A Articulation of facet joints
B Lamina
C Posterior surface of vertebral body

D Estimate of depth to epidural space
   Dotted line circumference of subarachnoid space

Figure 3.7 Ultrasound location of the epidural space

problem. Choosing a different space may also be helpful. The woman may be able to confirm the position of the mid-line. Ultrasound may be helpful in identifying the anatomical structures and the depth to ligamentum flavum (Fig. 3.7).

Difficulty in reaching the ligamentum flavum

This can usually be overcome by attention to the following:

- Try to imagine the angle of the spinous processes.
- Check the alignment of the needle. It should be central, in the interspinous space and in the mid-line.

Difficulty in advancing through the ligamentum flavum
Tough ligament

This is often found in sportswomen and very occasionally in a woman with a calcified ligament – a condition rarely present in women of child bearing age. A considerable degree of controlled pressure is required to broach a tough ligament, when doing so it must be remembered that the ligament is being pushed ahead of the bevel and so nearer to the dura.

Soft ligament

This may be found in obese or oedematous women. A soft ligament requires great care as there may not be a positive loss of resistance when the ligament is broached but rather a change of feel.

Puncture of the dura

This occurs when the epidural needle has travelled too far into the epidural space and punctured the dura leading to backflow of CSF. There is usually no doubt about the diagnosis. Further management is discussed in Chapter 11.

Difficulties in threading the catheter
The catheter will not thread out of the end of the needle

This may occur because the needle is not in the epidural space or the bevel of the needle is held within the ligamentum flavum thus obstructing the catheter (Figs. 3.5 and 3.6). Two manoeuvres can help:

- try advancing the needle a very small amount
- try turning the needle through 180°.

(NB These manoeuvres are associated with an increased risk of dural puncture.)

The catheter will not thread into the epidural space

When this occurs or when pain is produced on advancing the catheter, there is no alternative to removing needle and catheter *together* and starting again. The catheter must never be forced or withdrawn through the needle.

Blood in the catheter

The persistent presence of blood in the catheter should be assumed to be due to cannulation of an epidural vein. If the blood does not clear easily with saline and continues to be aspirated, there is no alternative to removing needle (if still in place) and catheter and starting again.

Cerebrospinal fluid in the catheter

If the fluid in the catheter is thought to be CSF, testing for the presence of sugar with a BM-Stix may help to resolve this as a small amount of glucose is normally present in the CSF. As a general rule, if there is any suspicion that the fluid in the catheter is CSF, the epidural should be abandoned and the woman should be treated as for a dural puncture (Chapter 11). If it is clear the epidural catheter is in the CSF, then consider using it as an intrathecal catheter (see Chapter 11).

Spinal and combined spinal epidural analgesia and anaesthesia

Spinal anaesthesia

Spinal anaesthesia is a technique where the dura (see Chapter 2) is deliberately pierced and local anaesthetic is injected directly into the cerebrospinal fluid (CSF). This is usually a 'one-shot' technique, although fine catheters are available for insertion into the CSF. The technique is simple to perform but requires meticulous attention to sterility. The potential for disaster is great if spinal anaesthesia is undertaken carelessly.

The advantages and disadvantages of spinal anaesthesia compared with epidural anaesthesia in relation to the clinical situation are summarized in Table 4.1.

Spinal anaesthesia in obstetrics can be particularly useful where the advantage of speed of onset outweighs the problems of hypotension and post-spinal headaches. The most obvious example is an emergency Caesarean section where the use of spinal anaesthesia may be the only means of avoiding a general anaesthetic. Spinal anaesthesia is also of benefit for short procedures in the perinatal period and in some circumstances in labour (see Chapter 8).

The main contraindications to spinal anaesthesia are as follows.

1. Contraindications to any regional technique:
   - patient refuses
   - sepsis at the site of insertion
   - operator not skilled in the technique.
2. Contraindications specifically to spinal anaesthesia:
   - raised intracranial pressure associated with cerebral tumour
   - any situation where a profound drop in blood pressure would be dangerous (for example some forms of heart disease)
   - hypovolaemia (the combination of hypovolaemia and the sudden sympathetic block caused by the spinal anaesthetic can produce a profound hypotension)
   - a procedure of indefinite duration.

Table 4.1 Advantages and disadvantages of spinal anaesthesia

Advantages	Disadvantages
Simple to perform as a 'one-shot' procedure	Lasts for a limited time
Fast onset of action: useful in emergency situations	Fast onset of sympathetic block • profound fall in blood pressure • adequate pre-load essential • prophylactic ephedrine advisable
Reliable (absence of anatomical variations that can cause problems with epidurals)	Less control than with epidural; therefore it can be difficult to adjust level of block
Needs small dose of local anaesthetic (e.g. 2.5 ml 0.5% heavy bupivacaine) • less risk of local anaesthetic toxicity compared with epidural	More nausea and vomiting than with epidural Post-spinal headache (6–16%)
Excellent surgical anaesthesia	Cannot be topped up for post-operative analgesia

Performing a spinal anaesthetic

There are many similarities between the method for setting up and performing epidural analgesia/anaesthesia and spinal anaesthesia. The method is described below with explanations of the main differences in technique.

Description and choice of spinal needle

As mentioned above, one of the disadvantages of spinal anaesthesia is the incidence of post-dural puncture headache. To minimize this effect much attention has been paid to the design of spinal needles (Fig. 4.1) and over time spinal needles have evolved. The traditional spinal needle was bevelled and sharp, allowing it to cut the dural fibres. As a rule the finer the needle the less is the incidence of post-dural puncture headache, but in practice spinal anaesthesia becomes technically more difficult with needles of 27 or 29 gauge as these bend easily and can be damaged during insertion. Also, with these tiny gauges, the positive sign of CSF flowing back out of the needles is very slow (up to 1 minute) and multiple dural puncture is possible as the operator repeatedly tries to demonstrate CSF. This damage to the dura may result in a CSF leak and hence a greater incidence of post-dural puncture headache than would have been expected. However, in experienced hands excellent results can be consistently obtained with a 29-gauge needle, but for the occasional user or a 'learner' a 24- or 26-gauge needle will be more reliable and easier to use, particularly in an emergency situation.

It has also been shown that the incidence of post-dural puncture headache can be further reduced if the bevel of the needle is introduced parallel to the long axis of the vertebral canal.

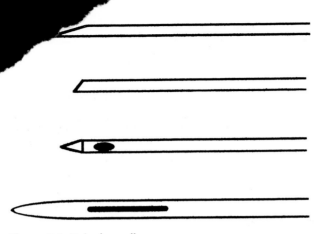

Figure 4.1 Spinal needles

A further development is the introduction of the 'pencil-point' (Whitacre) needle, which has its hole a few millimeters away from the end. This is designed to part the dural fibres rather than cut them, which is believed to reduce further the incidence of post-spinal headache. With this type of needle a larger gauge can be used (for example 24 gauge), which allows for greater ease of insertion. A refinement of this needle is the Sprotte needle, which has a more rounded tip than the 'pencil-point', that is similar to the shape of a bullet.

Equipment
- IV set, 16-gauge cannula and IV fluids
- sterile drapes
- gown, gloves, and mask and hat
- skin antiseptic
- spinal needle (size and choice as discussed above)
- filter needle
- syringe and needle for local anaesthetic infiltration
- swabs
- introducer (may be packaged with the spinal needle)
- local anaesthetic for the spinal (plus opiate if that is to be used)
- ephedrine and/or phenylephrine
- pump for intravenous administration.

It is of paramount importance that no infection or foreign matter is introduced into the CSF during the performance of a spinal. Unlike the epidural space, the dural space has no phagocytes or other defence mechanisms to protect the body against infection or debris such as particles of glass from an ampoule. Therefore a filter needle should always be used for this procedure.

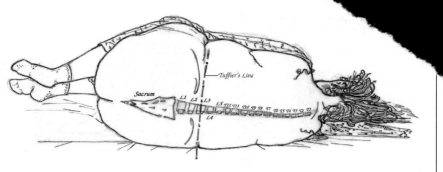

Figure 4.2 Bony landmarks with the patient in the left lateral position

Performing the spinal anaesthetic

Before commencing the spinal anaesthetic it is essential to ensure that the patient is monitored (electrocardiogram, blood pressure, pulse oximeter) and that a 16G cannula has been inserted. The patient should be preloaded with between 500–1000 ml of suitable fluid before the spinal anaesthetic is starting to work. The patient should then be positioned either sitting or lying in the left lateral position. The advantages and disadvantages of the sitting and lateral positions are in many ways identical to those for performing an epidural; however, there are two further points for consideration.

1. The area and level of the block will depend on the posture of the patient and the baricity of the local anaesthetic. When the patient is sitting, heavy bupivacaine 0.5%, which is denser than CSF, will gravitate to the sacral roots causing their innervation to be blocked first. Bupivacaine 0.25% as used for epidural anaesthetic is lighter than CSF and therefore will tend to rise above the site of introduction. With the patient in the left lateral position, heavy bupivacaine may produce a left unilateral block and the alteration of the fat distribution in pregnancy may result in gravitational flow of local anaesthetic to a higher spinal level (Fig. 4.2).
2. Local anaesthetic injected into the CSF has a very rapid action and can produce anaesthesia in 2–4 minutes. Thus it is essential to monitor the patient carefully with particular attention to the possibility of the development of sudden hypotension.

First the patient is positioned either:

- Sitting – with legs dependent and feet supported by a footstool and body curled over a pillow and two pillows placed at the head end of the table in readiness for transfer to the supine position with lateral tilt.
- Left lateral – curled on her left side as for an epidural.

The skin should then be cleaned with antiseptic as for an epidural and the sterile drapes placed on the patient. These should be positioned so that the can be palpated by the anaesthetist to assess the level of Tuffier's (see Chapter 3) and ensure that the spinal is performed below the level the termination of the spinal cord. Once an appropriate space has been identified e.g. L3–4 or 4–5 then local anaesthetic is infiltrated into the skin and deeper tissues. The introducer is inserted and then the spinal needle passed through the introducer. The introducer stabilizes the needle on its passage through the tissue layers to reach the dura. As the needle passes through the dura a slight give is felt, then the stillette is removed from the needle and the free flow of CSF is seen. Local anaesthetic is then injected into the CSF. The speed of injection of local anaesthetic will affect its spread. The injection should be steady, and barbotage (alternate aspiration of CSF and injection of local anaesthetic) should be avoided. The needle and introducer should be removed after the injection has been completed, and the patient should then be immediately helped into the wedged lateral position.

Local anaesthetics and any other drug introduced into the CSF must be sterile, free from glass particles or other debris and free from preservatives.

The most commonly used local anaesthetic in the United Kingdom is heavy bupivacaine 0.5% (bupivacaine prepared in glucose to produce a hyperbaric solution), which has an onset of action of 2–4 minutes and a duration of action of 75–120 minutes. It is now standard practice to mix the heavy bupivacaine with an opiate to improve the quality of the block. The most commonly used opiates are fentanyl 25 μg or diamorphine 250 or 300 mg.

It is worth repeating that careful monitoring is essential throughout this procedure and that the patient should never be left unattended. It is also prudent to warn the patient that the anaesthetic will act very quickly.

The physiological changes associated with spinal anaesthesia are largely the same as those for epidural analgesia, except that local anaesthetic injected directly into the CSF acts more quickly than with an epidural and therefore the effects are much more acute.

The most important of these effects is the potential for profound changes in blood pressure resulting from a sudden sympathetic block, and the following measures will act as a safeguard if carried out before the local anaesthetic is injected into the CSF.

- Preload with 500–1000 ml of Hartmanns solution.
- Phenylephrine is the drug of choice to maintain cardiovascular stability during Caesarean section and is usually administered as an infusion of 1 milligram per ml given at a rate commencing at 50 ml per hour then reducing the rate depending on the patient's blood pressure. It is essential that the infusion is primed and set ready to go as soon as the spinal is completed.
- Ephedrine is the drug that has traditionally been used and this should also be available. This can be given in 3 mg boluses to treat hypotension.

- Monitor the blood pressure preferably using an automatic monitor at least every minute for 5 minutes whilst the block is becoming established and thereafter at 10–15 minute intervals.
- Full resuscitation equipment should be readily available.

Problems associated with spinal anaesthesia

The following acute problems may be encountered in association with spinal anaesthesia.

1. Difficulty in siting the spinal needle. This may lead to multiple dural puncture when the needle is withdrawn and advanced as the operator attempts to establish that it is in the CSF. The result is a greatly increased chance that the patient will develop a post-spinal headache.
2. Pain during the insertion of the spinal needle. If this occurs due to the spinal needle touching the nerve fibres of the filum terminale then this may be transient, if the pain is severe or continues or is associated with the leg 'jumping' the spinal needle must be removed. If local anaesthetic is injected into a nerve this may cause serious neurological problems.
3. The block is too weak, uneven, or not high enough. Once the local anaesthetic has been injected and fixed its effect cannot be augmented or continued for a longer period by 'top-ups' as with an epidural. In this situation the anaesthetist is left with the choice of adding other methods of pain relief (for example Entonox or intravenous opiates) or abandoning the procedure.
4. The block is too profound. An ascending spinal block will cause a profound drop in blood pressure and respiratory difficulties, which may become sufficiently severe to warrant artificial ventilation of the patient and the administration of a general anaesthetic. The same basic principles of 'ABC' resuscitation apply as are described in detail for epidural analgesia/anaesthesia in Chapters 6 and 10.
5. The occurrence of hypotension is one of the major disadvantages of the technique and it should be anticipated and managed as described above.
6. Nausea and vomiting, often associated with hypotension, can be unpleasant for the patient and cause difficulties for both obstetrician and anaesthetist.

Post-spinal problems are similar to those described in detail for epidurals (see Chapters 10 and 11).

- post-spinal headache
- infection
- chemical contamination of CSF
- prolonged block.

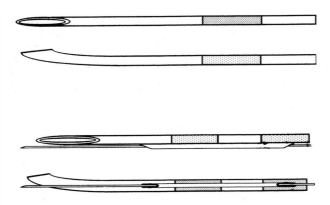

Figure 4.3 Epidural needles

The combined spinal epidural technique

This method involves performing a spinal anaesthetic and siting an epidural at the same time. The advantage of this combined technique is that it allows greater flexibility. A spinal anaesthetic can be used for rapid effect, following which an epidural catheter can be inserted to extend the block for continuing anaesthesia or post-operative analgesia.

There are three ways of performing this combined technique.

1. Use a standard Tuohy epidural needle to find the epidural space (as described in Chapter 3). Pass a long spinal needle across the epidural space, through the dura and into the CSF. For example a 120 mm 24G Sprotte needle can be passed through a 16G Tuohy needle.
2. Use a specially designed Tuohy needle with an end-hole to allow the smooth passage of a long spinal needle.
3. Use a specially designed Tuohy needle with a separate side channel to allow the passage of the spinal needle (Fig. 4.3).

What are the properties of the ideal epidural drug for use in labour?

In practice, the choice of drug for epidural analgesia in labour is based on a compromise between the desired effects and the side-effects. Drugs are now commonly used in combination to maximize the desired effects and minimize the side-effects. The ideal epidural anaesthetic drug for obstetric use would provide the following:

- safety to mother and baby
- excellent analgesia
- no effect on the normal progress of labour
- minimal effect on mobility.

Safety to mother and baby

The aim is effective analgesia with minimum side-effects to mother and baby. The potential effect of the drug on each system needs to be considered.

Central nervous system
The ideal drug will allow the mother to be awake (free from sedation, amnesia or confusion), relaxed and in full control of her labour. The baby should also be free from sedation during labour and after delivery so as not to interfere with feeding and bonding with the mother.

Cardiovascular system
The status of the maternal circulation determines the adequacy of the placental perfusion. A small drop in the maternal blood pressure may have a significant effect on the fetus, particularly if the placenta is compromised. The drug should ideally cause minimal cardiovascular depression even in the event of inadvertent intravenous administration.

Respiratory system
The effect of the drug on both the maternal and the neonatal respiratory system should be known and evaluated. Respiratory depression is not as

great a problem for the mother as for the neonate, which may have a reduced response to an increasing blood carbon dioxide concentration. Other effects on the maternal airways, such as bronchospasm are important.

General toxicity

The drug should be effective at a dose well below the amount that would cause toxic side-effects, i.e. it should have a high therapeutic index.

Ideally the drug should not accumulate in the body, and it should be useful for administration in repeated doses as is required for epidural top-ups. The incidence of non-specific irritating side-effects (for example nausea, vomiting, rashes, pruritis and retention of urine) should be low.

Excellent analgesia

The quality of analgesia provided is the most important property of the epidural anaesthetic drug. The analgesic or anaesthetic effect should be reliable, reproducible and dose related.

No effect on the normal progress of labour

The drug should not hamper the normal progress of labour.

Mobility

The drug should cause the minimum motor block. Women in labour wish to be ambulant, or when resting in bed they wish to have full use of their legs to allow a change of position at will. The ideal drug will allow the anaesthetist to provide selective analgesia thus enabling a pain-free labour whilst retaining motor power and sensation in the mother's birth canal and legs.

Unfortunately the 'ideal' epidural anaesthetic drug does not yet exist, but careful choice and educated management of the drugs currently available can limit the side-effects.

Drugs commonly used in epidural analgesia

The commonly available drugs used in epidural analgesia in the United Kingdom and Europe are local anaesthetics, the epidural opiates used alone or in combination with local anaesthetics and adrenaline used as an additive to local anaesthetics.

The choice of how and when to use each drug depends upon their individual properties, and these are discussed below under the following headings.

1. Local anaesthetics:
   - general pharmacology
   - placental transfer
   - metabolism
   - toxicity
   - allergy
   - tachyphylaxis (tolerance)
   - pharmacology of specific drugs.
2. Opiates:
   - mode of action of epidural opiates
   - choice of opiate
   - side-effects of epidural opiates.
3. Adrenaline:
   - use of adrenaline
   - the effect of adrenaline in reducing the systemic toxicity of local anaesthetics
   - the effect of adrenaline in increasing the duration of action of local anaesthetics
   - detection of intravenous administration
   - adrenaline preparations.

Local anaesthetics

General pharmacology

A nerve axon has membrane channels through which sodium ions (Na^+) can pass (Fig. 5.1).

In the resting state these channels are closed and the ionic balance between the internal and external part of the axon produces an electrical charge (potential difference) of around -70 mV. This ionic difference is maintained by the sodium pump, which maintains a higher concentration of Na^+ ions outside the cell compared with inside.

When the nerve is stimulated (depolarized) channels in the membrane briefly open allowing Na^+ ions to pass into the cell until a potential difference of $+20$ mV has been reached. This new potential difference stimulates (opens) adjacent channels leading to propagation of the signal (action potential) along the axon. It also causes potassium ions (K^+) to flow out of the cell. The sodium pump restores the balance resulting in repolarization of the nerve to its resting potential difference of -70 mV.

Local anaesthetic drugs block Na^+ movement through the ion channels of axon membranes. This effect requires the drugs to possess the property of being both water-soluble (ionized) and lipid-soluble (non-ionized). The water-soluble component allows the drug to transfer to the axon and the lipid-soluble component allows it to pass through the lipid membrane

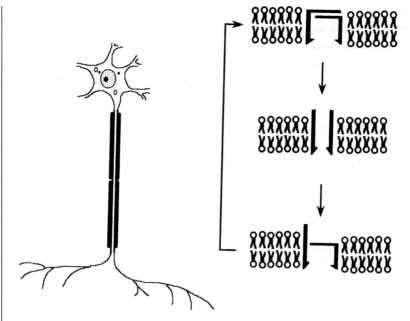

Figure 5.1 Sodium channel opening

covering the nerve, thus enabling the ion channels to be blocked (from within the nerve axon).

The proportion of lipid-soluble to water-soluble components of the drug determines its effect, as the rapidity of onset of action depends on the amount of lipid-soluble component available to the ion channel. The relative proportion of these components is governed by the ability of the drug to dissociate into ionized and non-ionized. The pK_a of the drug is the pH (acidity or alkalinity) at which 50% of the drug is ionized and 50% is non-ionized (that is, a drug with a pK_a of 7.4 will be 50% ionized and 50% non-ionized where the surrounding tissue has a pH of 7.4).

The properties of the local anaesthetic drug can therefore be represented schematically as follows:

lipid-soluble component active/ available (higher pH) water-soluble component inactive/ unavailable (lower pH)

All local anaesthetic drugs are weak bases and they have a pK_a greater than the physiological pH of 7.4: lidocaine has a pK_a of 7.87 and bupivacaine has a pK_a of 8.05.

The drugs are manufactured in a solution on the acidic (lower pH) side of the pK_a which has the effect of increasing water solubility and thus ease of transfer through the tissues at the time of injection. When the drug comes into contact with the more alkaline (higher pH) of tissue fluid the lipid-soluble component of the drug is released and travels through the nerve cell membrane to the axon where it stops the movement of Na^+, thus producing a conduction blockade.

If the tissues are acidotic, less local anaesthetic will be available in the axon and the conduction blockade will be less effective. A consequence of this is that more drug will be available in the tissues and in the circulation, which may increase its systemic toxicity.

A local anaesthetic drug's potency is determined by its inherent lipid solubility, the more soluble a drug is the less drug will have to be given for the same effect.

Local anaesthetic drugs have one further important property that governs their effect – the ability of the molecules of the drug to bind with plasma protein. This property will determine the amount of drug available in the systemic circulation, and so a high plasma protein binding capacity is associated with greater safety of the drug. (However, recent studies suggest that the importance of this may be less than initially thought.) The distribution and metabolism of the local anaesthetic and how this affects its action and toxicity is a dynamic situation, as illustrated in Figs. 5.2 and 5.3.

Placental transfer

Only the non-bound local anaesthetic in the circulation is available to cross the placenta. The amount that is available depends on the following factors:

- concentration gradient of the local anaesthetic across the placenta
- pH gradient across the placenta
- plasma protein binding of the local anaesthetic
- binding onto proteins with active transport mechanisms
- umbilical blood flow (which depends on placental perfusion).

All these factors taken together are part of a dynamic situation; hence the plasma protein-binding mechanism may not be the most important factor.

Metabolism

Currently used local anaesthetic drugs for epidural analgesia belong to the amide group. Amides are slowly metabolized by the liver and are mainly excreted unchanged in the urine. They are rapidly distributed in the body, and once lipid stores are saturated blood levels will rise due to the slow rate of breakdown and excretion.

Toxicity

When considering toxicity it is important to look beyond the nerve axon. The drug is not isolated in the epidural space but is absorbed into the systemic circulation and distributed throughout the body. This process is affected by the pharmacology of the drug(s) administered.

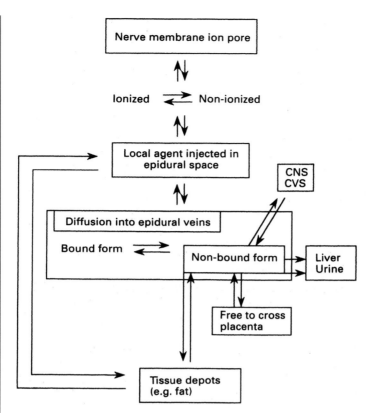

Figure 5.2 Distribution of local anaesthetic from the epidural space
(CNS: central nervous system; CVS: cardiovascular system)

The desired effect of local anaesthetics is to stabilize cell membranes to produce a conduction blockade, but this itself can lead to toxicity at the following sites.

- **At the site of action:** in obstetric use this will be in the epidural or intrathecal spaces. When correctly placed the effect is reversible and not toxic, but if the drug is accidentally injected into a nerve root permanent damage to that root is possible.
- **Distant to the site of action:** toxicity affects primarily the central nervous and cardiovascular systems.

Toxicity affecting the central nervous system
This central effect is mainly exerted on the brain and in particular in the medulla.

- **Brain:** toxicity causes excitation, which may result in convulsions and coma.

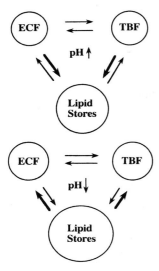

Figure 5.3 Effect of altered pH on the distribution of local anaesthetic (ECF: extra-cellular fluid; TBF: total body fluid)

- **Medulla:** the toxic effect is depression. As the medulla is the centre controlling respiratory and cardiovascular functions, these will be depressed.

Toxicity affecting the cardiovascular system
There is a direct effect on the heart, which is particularly sensitive owing to its large blood flow. Toxicity results in arrhythmias and cardiac arrest. An indirect effect is caused by depression of the medulla described above. The specific toxic effects of local anaesthetics are discussed in Chapter 10.

Allergy
There have been no well-documented cases of allergy to the amide group of local anaesthetics.

Tachyphylaxis
Tachyphylaxis is acute tolerance to a drug. In the case of local anaesthetics this results in a decrease in effect, a shorter duration of action and a poorer quality of analgesia. These effects become more pronounced with repeated doses of the drug.

Pharmacology of specific drugs
Table 5.1 shows data for some commonly used local anaesthetics.

Table 5.1 Pharmacology of commonly used local anaesthetics

Drug	pK_a	Protein binding	Onset	Duration
lidocaine	7.87	64%	fast	short
bupivacane (and levobupivacaine)	8.05	96%	slow	long
ropivacaine	8.10	95%	slow	long

Opiates

Mode of action of epidural opiates

Opiate receptors are present in the spinal cord and when opiates bind with these transmission of painful sensations is modified. The impulses from the painful organ (for example the uterus) are blocked in the spinal cord and thus are prevented from passing to the antero-lateral tract of the spinal cord. Therefore there is reduced transmission of pain signals from that organ to the thalamus or reticular awakening centre in the medulla.

The degree of binding of an opiate to these receptors in the spinal cord depends upon its lipophilic properties – the more lipophilic the opiate the better is the binding. An opiate that does not bind well with its receptors may leave sufficient in a 'free' state to be absorbed into the blood stream to exert systemic effects.

When opiates were first introduced to epidurals in obstetrics they were heralded as a means of producing excellent analgesia with minimal side-effects. Unlike local anaesthetics, there would be no risk of motor blockade or hypotension. In practice their usefulness in this application in isolation has been found to be limited. They are commonly used in combination with a local anaesthetic for labour or delivery and remain an excellent choice for post-operative analgesia. The theoretical advantages of this are that the side-effects from the local anaesthetic should be reduced and there should be a reduction in the motor block. A development of this principle is in the mobile epidural where the patient may remain ambulant with an epidural *in situ* (see Chapter 7).

Choice of opiate

As explained above, a lipid-soluble opiate should be chosen for use in the epidural space as this will bind more effectively to the spinal cord opiate receptors, and therefore will have fewer systemic side-effects. Morphine is less lipophilic than diamorphine or fentanyl and therefore will have a greater incidence of systemic side-effects.

The drug of choice in the UK for labour is fentanyl in a dose range of 25–50 µg. Additionally, epidural opiates have an established place in obstetrics in the following clinical situations.

1. **Management of perineal pain:** epidural fentanyl can abolish this pain when large doses of local anaesthetic have been ineffective in reaching the sacral roots.
2. **Shivering:** a small dose of epidural fentanyl may abolish this annoying side-effect of local anaesthetic.
3. **Caesarean section:** the use of opiates for Caesarean section is fully discussed in Chapter 12.

Side-effects of epidural opiates

Even in small doses, opiates introduced into the epidural space can have the following side-effects.

- Pruritus: this can be a distressing side-effect but has no serious significance.
- Respiratory depression: this results from a reduced ventilatory response to carbon dioxide and can be enhanced if other opiates (for example intramuscular pethidine) have been administered. For this reason a cautious approach is best in patients who have recently received systemic opiates. All patients receiving epidural opiates require careful observation.
- Nausea, vomiting and delayed gastric emptying.
- Urinary retention.

Adrenaline

Use of adrenaline

The addition of adrenaline to local anaesthetic solution for use in the epidural space provides the following theoretical advantages: a reduction in systemic toxicity, an increase in the duration of action of the local anaesthetic and detection of intravenous administration. In practice, the use of adrenaline creates problems that may outweigh these advantages. The main clinical use of adrenaline in obstetric epidurals in the UK is in enhancing the speed of onset of local anaesthetic, for example in Caesarean section (see Chapter 12).

The effect of adrenaline in reducing the systemic toxicity of local anaesthetics

The addition of adrenaline to the local anaesthetic solution causes local vaso-constriction in the epidural space. This limits the amount of local anaesthetic lost into the systemic circulation, thus reducing the possibility of systemic toxicity. The risk is that too much adrenaline in the epidural space may cause a spinal artery thrombosis, and this risk increases if the maternal blood pressure falls.

The effect of adrenaline in increasing the duration of action of local anaesthetics

In theory the vasoconstricting action of adrenaline in the epidural space should increase the duration of action of the local anaesthetic. In practice, this does not happen to a significant degree.

Detection of intravenous administration

An accidental intravenous injection of an adrenaline-containing solution will produce a rapid rise in heart rate and blood pressure. This effect can be used to advantage in test doses of local anaesthetic plus adrenaline to check the correct placement of an epidural catheter. In practice, this is difficult to assess (this is discussed in Chapter 3)

Adrenaline preparations

Adrenaline is manufactured in a 1% solution and is available in 1 ml ampoules containing 1 mg of 1:1000 adrenaline. Concentrations down to 1:200 000 are found to be clinically useful.

Bupivacaine and lidocaine are available with adrenaline in preprepared ampoules. These solutions also contain the antioxidant sodium metabisulphite, which reduces the pH of the solution and delays the onset of action of the local anaesthetic.

If adrenaline is freshly mixed with local anaesthetic solution at the time of use, the pH is not significantly altered. The vasoconstricting effect of the adrenaline contains the local anaesthetic in the epidural space without the penalty of reduced pH of the prepared solutions; thus the onset of action of the epidural block is shortened.

6 Physiological changes caused by epidural analgesia

Epidural analgesia is the most reliable form of pain relief in labour. Understanding the physiological changes produced by an epidural depends upon a full understanding of the physiological response to pain. This chapter is divided into two sections: the physiological response to pain; and the physiological changes produced by epidural analgesia (a) by relieving pain and (b) due to the epidural itself.

Physiological response to pain

The sensation of pain can usually be regarded as a warning that all is not well in that part of the body where it originates. The pain in labour arises from the uterus, the cervix and the birth canal, and it is visceral (that is secondary to the stretching of smooth muscle).

The pain threshold can be reduced because of fear and anxiety, both of which can be allayed in pregnancy and labour by the trust built up during antenatal preparation and parentcraft classes. Fatigue can reduce the pain threshold, and pain can cause fatigue. Therefore in labour the prevention of pain and fatigue depends upon a combination of effective management of labour and analgesia. This is also influenced by the fact that each woman will cope with the pain of labour differently, and each labour will be different.

As will be explained later in this chapter, the experience of severe pain can be harmful to both mother and baby, and so pain relief should be seen as an essential part of the good management of labour rather than as a luxury.

Pain pathways

Pain is transmitted via the visceral nerves by the slow conducting Aδ and C fibres from the uterus, and these nerves enter the spinal cord at T10–L1 via the dorsal nerve roots. These nerves then synapse in the substantia gelatinosa, and after ascending a few segments the fibres cross over and ascend further to become the lateral spinothalamic tract, which synapses in the thalamus. The pain impulses are then modified by the reticular activating system and the hypothalamus, and the painful impulses then reach consciousness in the

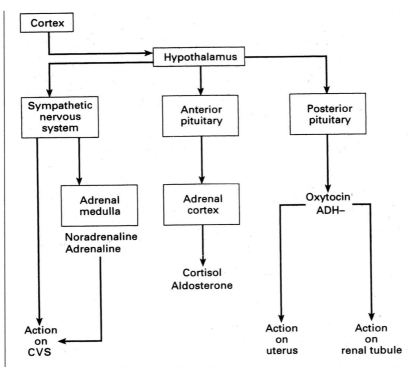

Figure 6.1 The widespread effect of pain on body systems (ADH: antidiuretic hormone; CVS: cardiovascular system)

cerebral cortex. The pain is then referred to the dermatomes supplied by the same nerve roots, i.e. the lower abdomen and back. Painful stimuli from the cervix, vagina and perineum are transmitted by the pudendal nerve to the 2nd, 3rd and 4th sacral roots.

The interaction between the cerebral cortex and the sympathetic and parasympathetic nervous systems in response to pain is complex. The effects of pain on the reticular activating system and the autonomic nervous system produce the physiological responses to pain. These responses can have far-reaching multisystem effects, as shown in Fig. 6.1. The far-reaching effects of pain illustrated in this diagram can best be described system by system.

Central nervous system

Pain, fatigue, fear and anxiety are often closely related, and they produce an arousal response in the central nervous system. If pain in labour is severe and/or prolonged, the woman may become distressed, irrational and exhausted to a degree where she is unable to cope.

Cardiovascular system

Pain exerts its effects on the cardiovascular system via the stress response mediated directly through the sympathetic nervous system and by the hormonal effects of noradrenaline and adrenaline secreted from the adrenal medulla. In the mother these effects increase the heart rate, stroke volume and contractility of the heart, which in combination with peripheral vasoconstriction result in an increased myocardial workload and oxygen consumption and decreased placental perfusion. The decrease in placental perfusion may be a significant problem where there is poor placental function. Women with high levels of circulating catecholamines have a higher incidence of abnormal fetal heart-rate patterns.

Metabolism

Pain stimulates the adrenal cortex to increase levels of cortisol and aldosterone in the body to produce the following metabolic effects:

- increase in protein catabolism
- hyperglycaemia
- decrease in insulin secretion
- sodium and water retention
- increase in serum potassium
- increase in mobilization of fat
- increase in ketone production.

The physical work of labour combined with the increased metabolic rate resulting from the sympathetic response to pain causes a metabolic acidosis. The metabolic consequences of a painful labour can therefore have deleterious effects on both the mother and fetus and the extent of this will depend on the severity of the pain and stress.

Respiratory system

During pregnancy there is an increased sensitivity to carbon dioxide that leads to a lower carbon dioxide level in the mother. Pain is associated with hyperventilation, which can result in an increase in the respiratory alkalosis of pregnancy and this may lead to vasoconstriction of the placental vascular bed and fetal compromise. This alkalosis is opposed by a corresponding metabolic acidosis, a condition already contributed to by uterine work.

Gastric emptying

Pain, distress and anxiety all inhibit gastric motility and therefore decrease gastric emptying. This increases the incidence of nausea and vomiting. The use of systemic opiate analgesia at this stage can exacerbate this problem.

Uterine function

Uterine contractions become uncoordinated in severe pain. This is often associated with a prolonged labour, dehydration and keto-acidosis.

Thus pain in labour may cause significant physiological effects, which are potentially harmful to both mother and fetus.

The physiological changes produced by epidural analgesia

The physiological actions of an epidural can be divided into those produced by relieving pain and those related to the epidural itself.

Physiological changes in response to pain relief

The physiological effects of pain relief are largely a negation of the effects of pain described in the previous section. The complete relief of pain that can be brought about by an epidural also removes stress with the following dramatic beneficial effects on the body systems.

Central nervous system
- A reduction in fear and anxiety levels.
- The ability to rest or sleep, thus preventing fatigue.

Cardiovascular system
- Abolition of increase in blood pressure and pulse rate due to pain.
- Reduction of stress and subsequent reduction of noradrenaline and adrenaline levels.
- Reduction in sympathetic nervous system activity, with a consequent improvement in peripheral circulation.
- Improved placental perfusion.

Respiratory system
- Hyperventilation abolished.
- Carbon dioxide levels return to normal for pregnancy.

Metabolic effects
- Metabolic acidosis reversed.
- Noradrenaline, adrenaline and cortisol levels reduced.
- Deranged glucose homeostasis corrected.
- Resolution of ketosis.

Gastric emptying
- Less vomiting.
- Approaches the 'normal' for pregnancy.

Uterine function
- Normal contractions can resume (uncoordinated uterine contractions can be associated with severe pain).

Physiological changes due to the epidural itself

Epidural analgesia produces excellent pain relief, but it has a marked effect on the sympathetic nervous system.

The local anaesthetic agent used in epidural analgesia acts in the epidural space to block the pain fibres but it also blocks the sympathetic nervous system. This effect is directly related to the amount of local anaesthetic administered. The increasingly standard practice of using low concentrations of local anaesthetic combined with an opiate for labour analgesia means that the sympathetic effect of the block is less. It is important that the sympathetic effects of epidural analgesia are not forgotten as they can be easily missed.

The sympathetic block of an epidural usually extends two segments above the sensory block. The effect of this will be most significant when the block is extended to the T4–T6 sensory level as may be required for Caesarean section. It is important to remember that the unblocked portion of the sympathetic nervous system is functioning normally and that activity from this portion will be reflexly increased in an awake, anxious patient.

The sympathetic block resulting from epidural analgesia has extensive physiological effects, which can be classified into three main groups:

- effects on the cardiovascular system
- effects on the endocrine system
- effects on temperature and shivering.

Effects of the sympathetic block on the cardiovascular system
The most important effect of the sympathetic block caused by epidural analgesia in clinical practice is on the cardiovascular system.

Effect on the heart
The sympathetic outflow to the heart is from T1 to T4–5, and if these segments are blocked the heart will be exposed to unopposed action of the vagus nerve. A sympathetic block up to this level is unlikely to occur in labour but may occur with an epidural for Caesarean section.

Unopposed vagal action on the heart produces a bradycardia, which should be treated with a sympathomimetic drug, such as ephedrine. A

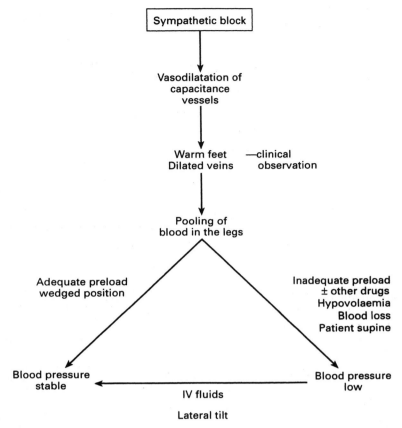

Figure 6.2 Effect of sympathetic blockade on the peripheral circulation

patient with a severe bradycardia caused by epidural analgesia may not be able to correct her cardiac output, and if venous return is coincidentally hampered by inferior vena caval compression (as may occur in the supine position) cardiac arrest may rapidly follow. This potentially fatal combination should be avoided or rapidly recognized and treated as follows if it occurs:

drop in blood pressure		place patient in full lateral tilt
		give intravenous fluid
+	URGENT TREATMENT	give oxygen (mask)
decrease in pulse rate		give ephedrine/atropine

Effect on the peripheral circulation

In the routine use of epidural analgesia for labour the sensory block does not usually reach above T10. Therefore the sympathetic effects will affect the peripheral circulation rather than the heart, as shown in Fig. 6.2. The extent of this sympathetic block will depend on the amount of local anaesthetic administered. This is the reason that with low dose mixtures the sympathetic effects of the epidural are seen less commonly. It is important that these effects are not forgotten as it is still routine practice for stronger solutions of local anaesthetic to be given for an instrumental or operative delivery (see Chapter 8).

Without an epidural the normal response of the cardiovascular system to supine hypotension caused by inferior vena caval compression is vasoconstriction of the blood vessels at the periphery of the **whole** body. The effect of this is to return blood to the central areas of the body that counteracts the drop in blood pressure. When an epidural is *in situ* the peripheral vasculature in the lower part of the body is prevented from vasoconstricting in response to hypotension by the coexisting sympathetic block. Therefore the presence of cold blue hands when the feet appear warm and well perfused should alert the clinician to relative hypovolaemia and to the need for more intravenous fluid.

The management of the cardiovascular effects of an epidural

The safe management of an epidural to avoid potential cardiovascular problems is based on two important principles:

- attention to **posture**
- prior administration of intravenous fluid – **preload.**

Posture

The routine use of uterine displacement whilst the woman is in bed should ensure that the weight of the gravid uterus is never allowed to impinge upon the major vessels. This is a general rule that becomes essential in the presence of epidural analgesia. This can be achieved by either by a 15° wedge or nursing the patient sitting or in the lateral position.

Without uterine displacement, blood pools in the legs as it is prevented from returning to the heart by the weight of the gravid uterus pressing on the inferior vena cava and the more turgid higher-pressure abdominal aorta allowing blood to flow to the legs. The result is that initially the patient suffers from a hypovolaemic faint, but with continuing pressure a cardiac arrest could occur. Therefore the first step in resuscitation in pregnancy should *always* be to displace the gravid uterus laterally before instituting other procedures (cardiac massage in the presence of an obstructed vena cava is useless as the heart will remain empty due to failure of return of venous blood from the lower half of the body). A further advantage of avoiding supine hypotension is that placental perfusion is maintained, thus preventing harm to the fetus.

Uterine displacement is discussed further in Chapter 7.

Preload

To compensate for the inevitable sympathetic block and consequent peripheral vasodilation of the lower limbs produced by an epidural, intravenous fluid is given immediately prior to the epidural to prevent hypovolaemia. This preload is given quickly under the following guidelines:

- 500 ml of crystalloid solution where the woman is in early labour and has previously been well hydrated
- 1 litre of crystalloid solution where the woman has been labouring for a long time and may be dehydrated
- 1 litre of crystalloid solution before a regional anaesthetic for Caesarean section.

The administration of crystalloid solutions in large volumes is not without its problems (for example, interference with the electrolytes in the neonate); therefore additional amounts should be given with care. Crystalloid is short lived in the circulation, about 3–5 hours. To reduce the amount of crystalloid used or where a quantity of crystalloid has already been given, colloid (for example, Haemaccel or Hespan) may be preferred. Colloids remain in the circulation for a considerably longer period than crystalloids.

Since vasodilatation is the major reason for the cardiac instability produced by a sympathetic block, the administration of a sympathomimetic drug such as ephedrine can be used to maintain a reasonable sympathetic tone and thus prevent or treat a drop in blood pressure. Ephedrine can be given as 3 mg boluses or as an infusion, and the rate of administration should be carefully titrated against the blood pressure (that is, give more if the blood pressure is low). An uncontrolled drop in blood pressure leads to maternal and fetal hypoxia, but equally an uncontrolled rise in blood pressure can lead to a reduced uterine blood flow.

In conclusion, a **moderate** preload combined with **careful** administration of ephedrine, with the patient always nursed with uterine displacement, will ensure a safely managed epidural where sympathetic block is a risk.

The woman in labour may maintain a normal blood pressure and pulse rate and look well even when a large fluid loss has occurred. In such cases epidural analgesia and sympathetic blockade may precipitate a disastrous drop in blood pressure. To avoid this possibility, all epidurals must have the following preconditions:

- intravenous access
- intravenous fluids
- lateral uterine displacement.

Other useful methods that can be employed to avoid hypotension are as follows.

1. **Raising the legs:** this may prove useful as an immediate additional measure in an emergency situation.
2. **Avoid sudden movement:** sudden movement, particularly in a woman prepared for Caesarean section, may precipitate a fall in blood pressure.

Effects of the sympathetic block on placental perfusion

Stress itself can decrease utero-placental blood flow, a factor that can be alleviated by epidural analgesia as long as the maternal blood pressure is maintained at normal levels. Therefore a carefully managed epidural can improve placental perfusion and fetal well-being.

Any alteration in the systemic blood pressure in the mother will produce an effect on placental perfusion as the uterine blood flow is proportional to the uterine perfusion pressure (the perfusion pressure is equal to the difference between the arterial pressure and the venous pressure).

Effects of the sympathetic block on the endocrine system

Stress due to pain or anxiety normally causes adrenaline secretion sufficient to stimulate gluconeogenesis, a rise in blood sugar levels, and ketoacidosis.

The sympathetic block resulting from an epidural has an effect on the endocrine system via the sympatho-hepato-adrenal axis thus preventing the hyperglycaemic ketoacidotic response to stress.

The efferent impulses to the adrenal medulla and liver involved in gluconeogenesis and release of adrenaline are T4–S5.

Effects of the sympathetic block on temperature and shivering

A slight increase in temperature or shivering are common side-effects of epidural analgesia, but the reasons for these are not entirely clear. One reason suggested is that sweating does not occur in those parts of the body affected by the sympathetic block (usually the lower limbs), but the cutaneous vasodilatation effect increases the rate of heat loss.

Therefore when the external environment is hot, absence of a sweating response may lead to a rise in body temperature. This slight rise in temperature is not related to infection and can be treated by simple measures, e.g. fan or paracetomol.

However, when the external environment is cold a shivering response may be more easily triggered. Shivering is not usually a problem, but where it becomes troublesome it can be treated with a small amount of epidural opiate (for example, fentanyl 25 μg).

This explanation does not accommodate the fact that shivering often occurs immediately after the injection of local anaesthetic solution into the epidural space and before the altered heat loss or gain could have occurred. To explain this phenomenon it has been postulated that this shivering reaction is due to stimulation of thermoreceptors in the spinal cord.

Epidural analgesia is a safe and effective method of providing analgesia in low-risk labour. It offers the best pain relief available, and if needed the epidural can be used for operative procedures that may be required. The evolution from traditional to low dose or 'mobile' epidural techniques has all but eliminated most of the problems traditionally associated with epidurals. It should also be remembered that women who develop problems during low-risk labour are more likely to request and receive epidural analgesia; this does not mean that the epidural is the cause of these problems.

Pain pathways involved in obstetrics

The practice of epidural analgesia in obstetrics requires an understanding of the relevant pain pathways. Pain in labour arises from the uterus and the birth canal. It varies in intensity and, although usually confined to the abdomen, a significant proportion of women experience pain in the back. Back pain can be particularly distressing to the mother and it is usually associated with an occipito-posterior position of the fetus.

During the first stage of labour the source of pain is mainly the uterus and cervix, but during the second stage pain from the birth canal becomes more significant. The pathways of pain in labour are illustrated in Fig. 7.1.

The relief of pain during the first stage of labour is achieved by placing local anaesthetic around the pain fibres in the segmental nerves T12 to L1–2. During the second stage (and in other instances – see Chapter 8) the pain fibres in the segmental nerves S2–4 should be blocked. The sensory impulses from the uterus are transmitted via the somatic nerves T12–L2, which are accompanied by the sympathetic innervation derived from T5–T12. The uterus has no parasympathetic innervation. The birth canal does not have a sympathetic innervation but is supplied by parasympathetic nervous system at the S2–S4 level. The parasympathetic nervous system plays a part in the reflex increase in oxytocin levels at full dilatation of the cervix (Ferguson's reflex).

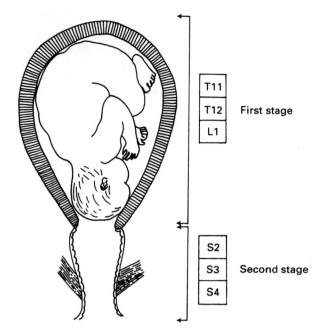

T11

T12 | First stage

L1

S2

S3 | Second stage

S4

Figure 7.1 Pain pathways in labour

The aim of continuous analgesia during labour

Choice of local anaesthetics

The aim of epidural analgesia is to provide pain-free labour with minimal side-effects (this topic is fully discussed in Chapter 5).

Local anaesthetic placed in the epidural space will affect all the modalities of sensation of the blocked segmental nerves to a greater or lesser degree. The effect of the local anaesthetic block should manifest itself in the following order:

- the sympathetic nerve fibres
- the pain fibres
- the proprioceptor and pressure nerve fibres
- the motor fibres.

This progression shows that in order to achieve analgesia a sympathetic block is inevitable. It also suggests that an adjustment of the dose of local anaesthetic can potentially produce analgesia without motor block. Various local anaesthetic agents are used to provide epidural analgesia, as has been discussed in Chapter 5.

The following factors govern the choice of the volume and concentration of local anaesthetic to be used in an epidural:

1. the greater the volume of the local anaesthetic, the greater is the spread of the block
2. the greater the concentration of the local anaesthetic, the greater is the density of the block with an increased chance of motor block.

Local anaesthetic can be injected into the epidural space as boluses or as a continuous infusion. The use of bolus top-ups is described in some detail below, and the place of epidural infusions is discussed later in this chapter.

Bolus administration of local anaesthetic

Bolus administration (commonly referred to as 'top-ups') is the traditional method of giving the local anaesthetic for an epidural in labour. Good analgesia can be achieved and maintained with this method by varying the volume and concentration of the local anaesthetic. However, the following points should be remembered.

- If the volume and concentration are too small analgesia is less likely to be successful. Frequent top-ups may be required, which is inconvenient for the midwife, the anaesthetist and the labouring mother.
- If the volume and concentration are too great an excessive block, extending over more segments than required, may be obtained together with an unwanted enhanced sympathetic effect. Higher volumes and/or concentrations increase the risk of exceeding toxic doses (see Chapter 5).

Management of labour with an epidural

Staffing considerations

The ideal staffing arrangement for labouring women requiring an epidural should be a midwife in constant attendance at all times. If there are staff shortages it is perhaps safer to limit the number of epidurals to the number of midwives available rather than expose the patient to any risks. In this situation the anaesthetist, the obstetrician and the senior midwife will place the women in order of priority for their epidurals.

The management of labour with an epidural is best linked to the three stages of labour.

The first stage of labour

The first stage of labour begins with the onset of regular uterine contractions causing cervical dilatation and ends when full dilatation of the cervix has occurred. The management of the epidural during this stage should have a systematic approach based on the following headings:

- analgesia
- posture
- monitoring of mother and baby
- checking the block.

Analgesia

The aim is that the labouring woman should be pain-free throughout the first stage of labour.

Posture

Attention to posture during the first stage of labour is an important part of management, which will not only improve the comfort of the patient but will also prevent potentially serious problems. The main points are avoidance of aorto-caval compression and of strain on the lumbo-sacral spine.

Avoiding aorto-caval compression

A labouring woman with epidural analgesia should be positioned so that the weight of the uterus does not impinge on the inferior vena cava or abdominal aorta. In effect this means that she should never lie flat on her back but should be nursed in either the full lateral position or with one buttock elevated by providing support with a pillow or a purpose-made wedge – a popular and practical solution. The wedge has an angle of 15° and is made of firm foam rubber covered with waterproof material. It is usual to place the wedge under one side of the mattress beneath the patient's buttock so as to tilt her laterally. The supine position is dangerous in epidural patients owing to the combination of aorto-caval compression and the sympathetic blockade effect of the epidural (that is there is no reflex vasoconstriction of the small blood vessels in the lower limbs to counteract this fall in blood pressure). The result is that the mother will faint and the baby will have a decreased placental perfusion. These effects are discussed more fully in Chapter 6.

Avoiding strain on the lumbo-sacral spine

An epidural has two effects that could cause strain on the lumbo-sacral spine:

- the normal sensation of pain or discomfort in the back or lower limbs will be diminished, allowing positions producing unnatural strain on ligaments to be endured
- motor blockade may leave the patient less able to mobilize.

Therefore it is an important part of epidural management that the anaesthetist and midwife ensure that the patient is encouraged to remain mobile and minimize inactivity.

If the mother wishes to stay in bed the best positions for avoiding ligament stress are full lateral or wedged positions with the head supported by pillows.

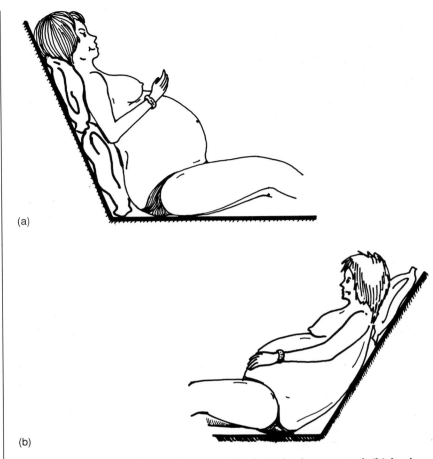

(a)

(b)

Figure 7.2 Sitting positions with an epidural: (a) back supported, (b) back unsupported

However, these are not popular resting positions as the woman is lying down and therefore appears to be an 'ill patient'. The wedged sitting position is more acceptable, but this requires meticulous attention to avoid ligament stress. Sliding into a 'banana shape' (Fig. 7.2b) is all too easy for the epidural patient who is unable to move her legs freely, and this can only be prevented by constant checking to see that the lumbo-sacral spine is well supported (for example, with a rolled-up towel) and that the wedge is in place under one buttock.

Monitoring of mother and baby

The monitoring of mother and baby should be visually charted on a partogram. The main features of the partogram are the regular recording of the following:

- heart rate, blood pressure and temperature
- fetal heart rate
- uterine contractions (strength and frequency)
- cervical dilatation (from regular vaginal examination)
- intravenous fluids
- urine output
- liquor (clear or meconium stained)
- drugs given (syntocinon, analgesia including top-ups, antacids and ranitidine, etc.).

All the above are part of standard obstetric management, but in a pain-free labour with an epidural greater care is needed to assess the strength and frequency of the uterine contractions and their effectiveness in producing cervical dilatation. In addition, the fetal heart should be monitored continuously using a cardiotocograph (CTG) as changes in placental blood flow can be exaggerated by the sympathetic block caused by the epidural. It should also be noted that there are many possible obstetric indications for the epidural where the condition of the baby may be compromised, for example prematurity and pregnancy-induced hypertension (see Chapter 8).

The routine monitoring of fluid balance is important, particularly in women with obstetric or medical problems. Gastric absorption is reduced during active labour, particularly if the woman is in pain or has been given opiates. Therefore significant dehydration and ketoacidosis usually occurs during prolonged labour. Dehydration is rapidly associated with ketoacidosis and with inefficient uterine action. Intravenous fluid should be administered where labour is prolonged. However, the administration of intravenous fluids is not without problems.

1. Fluid overload.
2. Hyponatraemia due to:
   - the anti-ADH (anti-diuretic hormone) effect of syntocinon administered in labour
   - the administration of a large volume of dextrose.
3. Interference with electrolytes in the neonate.

Therefore the correct amount of fluid, salts and dextrose to maintain haemostasis must be administered. The choice and amount of fluid depends upon the clinical condition of the patient and her fluid input and output. Crystalloid (electrolyte) solutions are most commonly used, although colloid solutions with their longer half-life and higher osmotic pressure in the circulation are indicated in certain clinical conditions, for example acute blood loss.

Blood pressure should be measured at periods of 5, 10 and 20 minutes after an epidural top-up, and also at any time when the condition of the patient causes concern (for example complaints of faintness or drowsiness or simply looking unwell).

Bladder sensation may be influenced by the epidural, resulting in difficulty with micturition. Therefore it is advisable to offer a bedpan to the patient before each epidural top-up and to encourage her to exert gentle pressure on the bladder to assist in the passage of urine. Evidence of retention of urine requires catheterization.

Prescribing top-ups

Epidural top-ups should be prescribed as follows:

- local anaesthetic type and concentration
- dose in millilitres
- maximum frequency of administration
- who is to administer the top-up
- any specific instructions
- action to take in case of problems.

Charting top-ups

Epidural top-ups should be routinely recorded as follows:

- time of top-up
- dose in millilitres
- local anaesthetic type and concentration
- efficacy
- blood pressure (at 5, 10 and 20 minutes)
- person who gave the top-up
- any problems.

Further comments on the recording of an epidural are given in Chapter 13.

Checking the block

The patient will be pain-free with a good epidural. However, it is good practice to check the epidural by assessing the sensory level and the motor block.

The **sensory level** can be checked by assessing the response to cold or to a pin-prick. Pin-prick is not recommended as it is difficult to perform and can leave the abdomen covered in tiny bleeding points. A cold stimulus (an ice-cube or ethyl chloride spray) is easier to use and is more reliable in giving an accurate result. The level of absence of sensation to cold touch should be recorded, together with a comparison of the left and right sides. During the first stage of labour an upper level of T10 (the umbilicus) and a lower level of L2–L3 (the thighs) should be maintained.

Assessing motor block prior to mobilization

The degree of **motor block** can be assessed using the following standard scale (Bromage):

    I. **complete** – unable to move feet or knees
   II. **almost complete** – able to move feet only
  III. **partial** – just able to move knees
  IV. **none** – full flexion of knees and feet.

Obviously, mothers who have a degree of motor block are not safe to mobilize out of the bed, and asking the woman to bend her knees as she steps out of bed is a useful way of assessing her ability to walk with the support of her partner or the midwife.

The second stage of labour

The second stage of labour begins at full dilatation of the cervix and ends with delivery of the baby.

Without epidural analgesia the onset of the second stage is heralded by a change in the character of the contractions as they become stronger, more frequent and more painful, accompanied by uncontrollable maternal expulsive efforts. Under the influence of epidural analgesia this is reduced or completely blocked, therefore pushing need not commence until the baby's head has descended into the birth canal.

A normal spontaneous delivery results unless it is impossible for an obstetric reason. It has been suggested that syntocinon infusions should be increased or introduced at this point if uterine contractions appear to be of poor quality.

The successful management of second stage labour with an epidural depends on the accurate diagnosis of the onset of full dilatation of the cervix by vaginal examination. Once full dilatation has been confirmed no action is required on the part of the mother or midwife until the mother feels a need to bear down or until the baby's head becomes visible on the perineum. Arbitrarily, some units encourage active pushing after one hour.

Epidural top-ups should maintain continuous analgesia throughout labour. Allowing the epidural to wear off at any stage is cruel to the patient who, having opted for an epidural, has a high expectation of a pain-free labour and delivery. The final top-up of local anaesthetic can be modified in dose and timing to limit the extension of the block to the sacral roots. There is no evidence to suggest that with modern 'low dose' epidurals altered sensation of the birth canal affects the expected outcome of a safe painless normal spontaneous delivery.

The third stage of labour

The third stage of labour lasts from delivery of the baby to delivery of the placenta and may include suture of the episiotomy or tear. The delivery of the placenta does not need additional analgesia unless there is a retained placenta that requires manual removal. Analgesia from the epidural should cover suturing the episiotomy or tear and a top-up may be necessary specifically for this purpose, particularly if the tear is extensive. See Chapter 8.

Who should give the top-ups?

The first top-up of the epidural should always be given by the anaesthetist who will at the same time check that the epidural is effective and safe. Thereafter top-ups may be given by the anaesthetist or delegated to a midwife who should be certified as having attended special tuition on the technique of epidural analgesia. The importance of teaching midwives and regarding them as part of the team is fully discussed in Chapter 13.

The involvement of the midwives in epidural analgesia is the linchpin that guarantees a smooth-running epidural service and gives the labouring woman the best chance of remaining pain free throughout her labour. In a busy unit the time taken to summon the anaesthetist may be long enough to allow the epidural block to wear off before the repeat top-up is given. However, it remains the anaesthetist's responsibility to manage the epidurals and to be readily available in the delivery suite to deal with problems.

Topping up the epidural

The first epidural top-up dose should be administered by the anaesthetist; subsequent doses may be delegated to the midwife.

Step-by-step guide to topping up an epidural

1. Check that the intravenous fluid is running, and that additional intravenous fluid is readily available should it be required.
2. Check that the patient has emptied her bladder recently and if she has not, offer a bedpan.
3. Wash your hands.
4. Check the prescription:
   - DRUG
   - CONCENTRATION
   - VOLUME.

It is advisable to check the drug with a colleague before administration.

5. Check the position of the epidural catheter by gentle aspiration – a safeguard against subsequent accidental intravenous or intrathecal injection of local anaesthetic. There should be no free aspiration of fluid or blood. This test (if negative) should not lead to complacency as problems can still occur. If there is any doubt, call the anaesthetist.

6. Posture:
   • check the instructions given by the anaesthetist
   • make sure that the patient is wedged.

7. Giving the top-up:
   • **When:** The local anaesthetic should be given between contractions, again to allow an even spread of the solution.
   • **How:** The local anaesthetic should be given slowly, for example 10 ml over 30 seconds. If the injection is given too quickly, a patchy block or excessive spread of the block may occur.

8. Monitoring: the patient should be continuously attended throughout the 20–30 minutes it takes for the local anaesthetic to bind to the tissues and take effect so that any adverse effects can be observed such as pallor, faintness, twitching or difficulty in breathing. Blood pressure should be measured at 5, 10 and 20 minute intervals and at any time that the patient feels unwell.

9. Analgesia should be complete within 20 minutes. If it is not, the extent of the block should be reassessed.

10. Documentation: details of the top-up and its effects should be recorded as discussed in Chapter 13. (An example chart is included in Appendix H.)

Any problems with an epidural top-up should immediately be dealt with by general measures:

• give oxygen via a face mask
• check that the patient is correctly positioned (lying horizontal, full lateral, wedged)
• increase the rate of infusion of intravenous fluids
• the midwife should call for help.

The anaesthetist will assess the nature of the problem to exclude the following:

• supine hypotension
• accidental intrathecal injection
• accidental intravenous injection of local anaesthetic.

These are dealt with in Chapter 10.

Epidural infusions and patient-controlled epidural analgesia

Local anaesthetic solutions can be administered into the epidural space by continuous infusion rather than by bolus top-ups or by a combination of the two. Comparison of the disadvantages of these methods highlights their differences and illustrates why infusions may be preferred in some instances.

Disadvantages of bolus top-ups of epidurals

• Intermittent pain, which is particularly liable to occur where a midwife or anaesthetist is not readily available to administer the local anaesthetic.

Disadvantages of continuous infusion of epidurals

• It takes longer to set up and maintain a steady state; therefore an infusion is useful only if labour is not too advanced.
• A safe and reliable volumetric pump for epidural use is required.

Each obstetric unit will develop its own preference for one or other method of giving epidurals – bolus top-ups or continuous infusions. Where there are few midwives trained to carry out top-ups, infusions may have advantages.

Method for setting up and monitoring continuous infusion

Local anaesthetic preparation
An epidural infusion is usually maintained via a volumetric pump connected to the epidural catheter using a high volume, low concentration of local anaesthetic, for example 10–20 ml/hour of bupivacaine 0.1% + fentanyl 2 μg/ml. The rate of delivery of the infusion should be set by the anaesthetist.

Monitoring

Clear instructions should be given by the anaesthetist to the midwife, and should include the following:

• regular measurement of blood pressure and pulse rate (for example every 30 minutes)
• a record of the level of altered skin sensation (to cold or pin-prick) with a set upper limit (for example T10)
• advice to switch off the pump if the block becomes too extensive.

Patient-controlled epidural analgesia

A development of the technique of epidural infusion is the use of patient-controlled epidural analgesia (PCEA), which may allow the labouring woman to have more individual control over her pain relief. Light compact pumps about the size of a personal stereo are now available, which are easy to programme and can be carried by the woman in a small shoulder bag.

The success of PCEA depends upon the following criteria.

• The epidural should be inserted early in labour before pain has become intrusive and to give the woman time to gain confidence in her use of the pump.

Method

The monitoring should be similar to that for a conventional epidural as described earlier in this chapter, although in practice we have found that the patient's blood pressure remains remarkably stable and measurement every 30 minutes is sufficient.

A commonly used example: fentanyl and bupivacaine mixture

• An epidural infusion is set up with a mixture of 2 µg/ml fentanyl plus bupivacaine 0.1%.
• The infusion is connected to a PCEA pump, as above.
• The pump is set to deliver 4 ml/hour continuous epidural infusion or a 3 ml bolus, as required (with a 10 minute lock-out time).

Our experience to date with current 'low dose' techniques is that all the labouring women have been sufficiently mobile to sit in a rocking chair, to help themselves onto a bedpan and to change their position at will. Many are able to walk around and to adopt alternative postures for delivery.

Postpartum

After delivery the epidural catheter is removed and once full strength has returned to the woman's legs mobilization can be unaided. It is also important to ensure that bladder function returns to normal and that the bladder is being emptied fully.

Many women go home six hours after delivery and some of these women may have had an epidural. It is advisable to have a leaflet for these women to take home with them informing them of the common side-effects, for example post-dural puncture headache, and a telephone contact with the obstetric anaesthetic team if they are worried.

Normally all women should be followed up after an anaesthetic intervention and any problems will be picked up on these routine visits.

Management of regional block for obstetric problems

The anaesthetist is an essential part of the team managing women with obstetric problems. Obstetric problems can be broadly divided under three headings.

- Problems that are recognized antenatally
- Problems that develop intrapartum
- Problems that present postpartum

Good analgesia or anaesthesia as provided by an epidural or spinal is an essential part of the safe and controlled management of these women. Good communication with the anaesthetist should enable proactive involvement as there are few problems that develop without warning.

Antenatal

The following conditions should be recognized antenatally and may require epidural analgesia as an integral part of their management.

- Breech
- External cephalic version for breech presentation
- Twins
- Vaginal birth after Caesarean section (VBAC)
- Pre-term labour, including cervical cerclage and rescue suture
- Pre-eclampsia
- Intra-uterine growth retardation
- Intra-uterine death or termination of a non-viable fetus.

Breech

A significant number of women will have a planned Caesarean section, particularly if they are primiparous, as the recent randomized controlled study on primiparous vaginal breech delivery has shown that Caesarean section is the mode of delivery of choice at term. Therefore there will be few women who will now choose to have a vaginal breech delivery. A breech presentation carries a risk of Caesarean section, which is a strong indication for epidural analgesia for all breech labours. Epidural analgesia offers great advantages in a vaginal breech delivery by combining good operative conditions with an awake, cooperative mother, therefore promoting a safe controlled delivery.

The anaesthetist should be called for the delivery of the breech in good time to assess the block and to top-up the epidural as if for an instrumental delivery. The ideal is that the woman should retain some urge to push, but that she should have sufficient analgesia for a painless delivery including the application of forceps to the aftercoming head. This ideal is difficult to achieve and requires the close attention of the anaesthetist throughout labour, particularly during the second stage.

Breech deliveries are unpredictable, and an assisted breech delivery may suddenly turn into a breech extraction with a great deal of manipulation, for example Loevset's manoeuvre for the delivery of the shoulders and arms.

Planned vaginal delivery of a breech presentation requires careful assessment and is best approached by considering primiparous and multiparous women separately.

For those primiparous women in whom a vaginal breech delivery is planned there are several points that should be taken into consideration.

1. Where a long, slow labour occurs, this is in itself an indication for an epidural.
2. With an epidural *in situ* there is a tendency for the woman to reach full dilatation of the cervix without the urge to push. With careful management of the epidural during the second stage of labour it should be possible to spare the sacral nerve roots, thus preserving the urge to push.
3. Less commonly, a primiparous woman will experience the urge to push before the cervix is fully dilated. In this situation selective blocking of the sacral nerve roots up to the point of full dilatation of the cervix will inhibit the breech being involuntarily pushed through an undilated cervix.
4. Breech delivery is often an operative procedure and therefore requires a well topped-up epidural, preferably with the anaesthetist in attendance.
5. About half of women who have commenced a labour with a breech presentation will end up with delivery by Caesarean section. An epidural already *in situ* can be used to provide anaesthesia for surgery, removing the need for general anaesthesia and its attendant risks.

The management of an epidural is simpler in the multiparous woman.

The multiparous woman labours more efficiently than the primiparous woman and she will usually have no difficulty in pushing at the onset of the second stage of labour. However, she may develop an uncontrollable desire to push before full dilatation of the cervix therefore the epidural should be sited in sufficient time to achieve a good block of perineal sensation so that the urge to push can be abolished until full dilatation of the cervix has occurred.

A low-dose spinal as part of a combined spinal epidural (CSE) block is often the regional analgesic of choice, since the spinal component of the block will give good perineal analgesia without motor block (see Chapter 7). A spinal injection of 1 ml of 0.25% bupivacaine and 25 µg of fentanyl will usually achieve excellent analgesia and abolishes the uncontrollable desire to push the baby out through an undilated cervix. The CSE can be placed using a needle-through-needle technique where the woman is reasonably calm and cooperative. If the woman is 'out of control' then the anaesthetist may choose to do a single-shot spinal as the safest option then return to place the epidural when the woman is calm.

External cephalic version for breech presentation

External cephalic version for breech presentation is offered to women whose baby presents as a breech. Usually this procedure is carried out without analgesia or anaesthesia, though in a small number of cases the anaesthetist may be asked to be involved. This is either to stand by if the fetus becomes compromised during the external cephalic version, or to provide analgesia to facilitate the version.

Twins

The main indication for an epidural arises from the problems that are often associated with delivery. These are mainly due to malpresentation of the second twin, for example breech, as discussed above. After the delivery of the first twin the position of the second twin is unpredictable and urgent Caesarean section or version (internal or external) may be required. The anaesthetist should be closely involved with a twin labour and should be on hand to supervise the final top-up. It is essential that the epidural be topped up before delivery of the first twin to give a block to an adequate level (T8). In the absence of epidural analgesia an urgent general anaesthetic may be required to enable delivery of the second twin.

There is always the possibility of delivery by Caesarean section and good epidural analgesia and the active involvement of the anaesthetist as part of the team at delivery should avoid the need for an urgent general anaesthetic.

Other points to consider in a twin pregnancy are as follows:

- increased risk of Caesarean section
- larger gravid uterus will increase the risk of supine hypotension
- increased incidence of prematurity
- increased incidence of pre-eclampsia.

For all the above reasons antenatal discussion of the benefits afforded by epidural analgesia in twin pregnancy is essential, and will allow the epidural to be sited in good time.

Vaginal birth after Caesarean section

Depending on the reason for their previous Caesarean section the incidence of a Caesarean delivery in this labour may be as high as 50%. Therefore an epidural sited for labour analgesia should be available to be topped up in the event of a Caesarean delivery. These women have a scar on their uterus and need careful monitoring throughout labour. Scar dehiscence causes significant morbidity and mortality in the mother and baby. The use of an epidural in the presence of a scar on the uterus has been controversial in the past, as it was felt that the pain associated with dehiscence of the uterine scar would be masked by the epidural. In fact the pain of a ruptured uterus breaks through the epidural block.

The whole team looking after the labouring mother must be vigilant and aware of the warning signs of uterine rupture. These are:

- scar pain and tenderness
- vaginal bleeding
- poor progress in labour
- fetal heart abnormality including acute fetal distress
- maternal collapse.

Scar pain will break through the epidural analgesia. It is important that the anaesthetist does not embark on topping up the epidural with a stronger and stronger solution without looking at the woman as a whole, and the character of the pain that may be present in between contractions as well as the fetal heart rate trace. If in doubt the obstetrician should be involved early. Uterine dehiscence may also occur in the absence of a scar on the uterus.

Pre-term labour, including cervical circlage and rescue suture

There are women whose baby needs to be delivered early for a fetal or maternal cause, and those where the woman goes into premature labour. With careful antenatal monitoring it may be decided that a baby is not going to benefit being in utero any longer and on the balance of risks and benefits delivery should be expedited; this may be for maternal or obstetric reasons. In these situations the anaesthetist should be an integral part of the decision-making as to mode of delivery. A detailed discussion of the problems that may arise, for instance, when the mother has severe heart disease is outside the remit of this book. Delivery is either by planned Caesarean section or induction of labour, and a regional block in the form of analgesia is an integral part of the management of these often complex clinical scenarios.

Premature labour causes everyone a great deal of anxiety and this needs good communication between all members of the team looking after the woman and her baby, and most importantly good communication with the mother to be and her family. It is always difficult to know when premature labour should be declared inevitable, and there is often a reluctance to discuss 'what if this labour is inevitable' and to involve the anaesthetist in the management of pain, ideally with epidural analgesia even if the labour stops. An epidural in abolishing pain will reduce stress and may help in the management of these women. Often the discussion of analgesia is rushed and suboptimal without adequate discussion of the risks and benefits. It is obvious that a compromised immature fetus would benefit from regional analgesia or anaesthesia being administered to the mother rather than the stress of pain or sedative effects of opiate analgesia.

Women with recurrent mid-trimester pregnancy loss may be offered cervical cerclage, and this can safely be performed under spinal anaesthesia aiming to achieve a block to T10. In the situation of an impending premature labour diagnosed by ultrasound demonstrating that the length of the cervix is shortening, a rescue suture may be considered. For this procedure spinal anaesthesia is suitable, though the block needs to reach up to around T6 and the patient needs to be able to tolerate a head-down tilt to facilitate the surgery.

Pre-eclampsia

Pre-eclampsia is a complication affecting 5–9% of pregnancies. It incorporates a spectrum of illness varying from mild hypertension, with or without proteinuria and oedema, to fulminating pre-eclampsia progressing to eclampsia with fits, cardiovascular catastrophes and renal failure. It is a disease that may result in multi-organ failure and death.

A multidisciplinary team approach is essential, with careful monitoring of all parameters to ensure that these women are managed safely. The most severe cases require a coordinated and intensive management by the obstetrician, the midwife, the anaesthetist and the paediatrician.

Epidural analgesia is often an integral part of the management of labour in pre-eclampsia. Good analgesia as provided by an epidural is needed for labour, particularly when labour is induced to prevent an additional rise in blood pressure in response to pain in the already hypertensive woman. The vascular bed in these women has an increased sensitivity to exogenous and endogenous catecholamines, and epidural analgesia helps to smooth out the peaks and troughs in the blood pressure allowing easier control. Placental perfusion is improved by well-managed epidural analgesia, and this can be important as the placenta flow is often compromised. The physiology of the above changes is explained in Chapter 6.

Before an epidural is sited in a woman with pre-eclampsia it is essential to do a full blood count. A falling platelet count may occur in pre-eclampsia and may be associated with bleeding, and this may manifest itself as a part of the HELLP syndrome (haemolysis, elevated liver enzymes, low platelet count) or disseminated intravascular coagulation (DIC). Close monitoring of the blood haematology and biochemisty is essential for these women. The platelet count is recommended as a guide as there is not yet a consensus on which clotting test gives the most reliable results, although a coagulation screen should be in the normal range. Bleeding time may be measured, and a time greater than 11 minutes should be a contraindication to epidural analgesia. Some units have thromboelastography (TEG) available to them and this may be the most reliable test for blood coagulation for these women prior to epidural analgesia. The risks of bleeding into the epidural space must be balanced against the benefits of epidural analgesia for each individual woman, though the following will act as a guideline.

- Platelet count is greater than 100×10^9/litre, proceed with the epidural.
- Platelet count is less than 100×10^9/litre (but greater than 80×10^9/litre), do a full coagulation screen and if this is normal proceed with the epidural.

There is increasing evidence that it is safe to site an epidural with a platelet count of 80×10^9/litre though this should be a consultant anaesthetic decision. If bleeding time is readily available (normal bleeding time is 10 minutes or less) or TEG, then they can be used as part of the clinical management for these women.

The epidural should be sited only once coagulopathy has been excluded and managed with a low dose of local anaesthetic, so that cardiovascular stability including placental perfusion is maintained.

In the absence of clotting problems in pre-eclampsia, epidural analgesia should be considered an integral part of the 'intensive care' input of the anaesthetist in such cases.

Intra-uterine growth retardation

Some babies become compromised in utero. It may be necessary to deliver these babies early if fetal ultrasound monitoring shows that that the baby is compromised. There are many reasons for a baby to be poorly grown and these may be obstetric with poor placentation, or maternal where the woman has an inter-current medical condition (e.g. cardiac disease). These babies may not tolerate labour and will need to be carefully monitored and often need to be delivered by Caesarean section.

If labour is induced, epidural analgesia should be an integral part of their management for the following reasons:

- to provide a pain-free and therefore stress-free labour
- to provide a slower second stage leading to a less precipitate delivery
- to ensure optimal placental perfusion
- to avoid the necessity for giving opiates or nitrous oxide to the mother, so that the neonate is free of sedative drugs in its circulation at birth.

There is also an increased chance of requiring intervention, for example fetal blood sampling, instrumental delivery or Caesarean section. If the baby needs to be delivered by Caesarean section then the epidural is available to be used for anaesthesia.

Intra-uterine death or termination of a non-viable fetus

The occurrence of an intra-uterine death or a grossly abnormal fetus is a very sad and emotional time for all concerned, and particular expertise and understanding will be called upon from the whole team. This traumatic event can be soothed by offering the woman the best analgesia available for the chosen method of delivery of the fetus, and this will often be achieved by an epidural. Patient-controlled analgesia with an opioid or sedation may also have a part to play in managing a delivery that is as comfortable and stress free as possible. If the intra-uterine death occurred more than a week before labour the presence of DIC should be excluded prior to epidural analgesia. A patient information leaflet should be provided so that the woman knows what analgesic options are available to her before admission to the delivery suite.

Intrapartum

The intrapartum management of obstetric problems that develop during labour will be discussed:

- slow progress of labour with tired mum
- need for fetal blood sampling (FBS)
- induction and augmentation of labour
- occipto-posterior position and other malpresentations
- instrumental delivery
- ventouse and lift-out forceps delivery
- rotational forceps delivery
- trial of instrumental delivery.

The first two in the above list are indications for epidural analgesia and the management of the epidural for labour is routine. Induction of labour with prostaglandins or oxytocin may give rise to a long, tedious and painful labour. The management of the epidural where the baby is in the occipito-posterior position and the management of instrumental delivery will be described in more detail.

Induction and augmentation of labour

Augmentation of labour with oxytocin should also be considered as an indication for epidural analgesia because a woman who has coped well with the pain of 'normal' labour contractions may not tolerate the enhanced contractions produced by the oxytocin. Also, women whose labour has been augmented are confined to bed and are therefore less mobile and less able to cope with pain. Once committed to delivery the epidural should be in place and working before the oxytocin infusion causes additional pain or distress. A slow and painful labour may be a marker for a dysfunctional labour and epidural analgesia should be seen as an integral part of the management of that labour. Often repeated fetal scalp blood sampling is required to monitor fetal well-being.

Occipito-posterior position and other malpresentations

The woman labouring with an occipito-posterior (OP) position is often distressed with back pain. These labours are often prolonged and result in ketoacidosis and incoordinate uterine action, leading eventually to maternal distress and emergency Caesarean section. The analgesia offered by an epidural can break the cycle of pain and distress, allowing labour to progress normally.

The only disadvantage of an epidural in an OP labour is that the abolition of pain and sensation in the pelvic floor and perineum may relax the pelvic floor musculature, thus inhibiting the normal rotation of the baby's head from posterior to anterior. This in turn may increase the necessity for rotational (Kielland's) forceps or ventouse delivery (see below).

When setting up an epidural in this situation it is advisable to give a total of 20 ml of bupivacaine 0.1% with 2 μg/ml of fentanyl as the first top-up dose, and to place the woman in the semi-recumbent position (remember the wedge).

Inadequate analgesia in an OP position is not acceptable as it leaves the woman with significant perineal pain or discomfort, which can give her an uncontrollable urge to push on an undilated cervix. Persistent perineal pain can be eased with the addition of a larger volume of the low dose solution, a small volume of stronger local anaesthetic or epidural fentanyl.

At full dilatation of the cervix in an OP position the epidural should be kept topped up to allow time for rotation of the baby's head. Once the head descends into the birth canal (in the OP or occipito-anterior position) the second stage of labour can be managed normally.

In a persistent OP position with failure of descent of the head despite adequate maternal effort the epidural should be checked with a view to providing analgesia for a forceps delivery (see below).

The CSE has a place in providing analgesia for these women and may provide better perineal analgesia from the onset without the development of a motor block. There is clinical evidence to support this but this is not borne out in randomized controlled trials (RCTs).

Instrumental delivery

Epidural analgesia should provide excellent analgesia and operating conditions for an instrumental delivery with the advantage of an awake and cooperative patient. The management of the epidural will depend on the type of instrumental delivery.

Ventouse and lift-out forceps delivery

These are performed when the baby's head has descended well into the birth canal. The most common obstetric indications for this procedure are delay in the progress of the second stage of labour caused by malposition, reduced maternal effort or maternal exhaustion and fetal distress. Unless there is a reason for urgent delivery, there is usually time for the midwife or anaesthetist to top up the epidural to provide good analgesia for the delivery.

The dose of local anaesthetic required for the top-up is usually 10 ml of bupivacaine 0.5% (depending on the time and dosage of the previous top-up) or 10 ml of 2% lignocaine with 1 in 200 000 adrenaline. This should produce effective anaesthesia for the forceps delivery after 10–15 minutes. It is essential to check the block before delivery paying particular attention to the perineum. For this purpose the block should extend from T10–S4. The obstetrician may need to infiltrate local anaesthetic for an episiotomy if the perineum is not adequately anaesthetized. It is important to remember to maintain lateral tilt with a wedge when the patient is put into the lithotomy position for a forceps delivery.

Rotational forceps delivery

Rotational forceps delivery is a technique for rotating the baby's head from the OP or occipito-transverse position to the occipito-anterior position before delivering the head into the birth canal and following on with a lift-out forceps or ventouse delivery. Depending upon the judgement of the obstetrician, the procedure may take place in either the delivery room or the operating theatre. Where there is doubt as to the ease of delivery and a possibility of proceeding to Caesarean section is entertained, a trial of forceps in theatre will be the choice.

For a straightforward rotational forceps delivery the epidural block does not need to be as profound as that for a trial of forceps, and so anaesthesia is as for lift-out forceps above.

Trial of instrumental delivery

When a trial of instrumental delivery has been decided upon this should take place in the operating theatre, the epidural should be topped up as for a Caesarean section with a block covering T4–S5 (see Chapter 12). When in doubt it is wise to plan for a Caesarean section rather than be faced with the need for an emergency general anaesthetic.

If the patient does not have an epidural then regional anaesthesia can be provided as for an emergency Caesarean section (see Chapter 12)

Postpartum

- Retained placenta
- Postpartum surgical procedures.

Retained placenta

Manual removal of the placenta can be safely performed under regional anaesthesia. Indeed, it is the recommended anaesthetic in the absence of significant blood loss as general anesthesia will inevitably mean that the woman is separated from her baby and can also be associated with unwanted uterine relaxation and further blood loss. However, if there is an associated significant postpartum haemorrhage, a general anaesthetic may be more appropriate. Therefore assessment of blood loss and correction of hypo-volaemia is necessary before a regional block is considered.

The regional block should extend from an upper level of T8 to a lower level of S2–S4. This can be obtained either from topping up an epidural already *in situ* or from a spinal inserted specifically for the procedure. When topping up an epidural lignocaine 2% with 1 in 200 000 adrenaline (10–20 ml) is the local anaesthetic of choice as it has the advantage of acting more rapidly than bupivacaine, allowing speedier mobilization of the patient afterwards.

For spinal anaesthesia there is no current consensus for the amount of local anaesthetic needed and doses vary between 1.5–2 ml of heavy bupivacaine with 25 μg of fentanyl used to provide a satisfactory block.

Postpartum surgical procedures

The performance of postpartum surgical procedures (for example third-degree tear, cervical laceration or evacuation of a vaginal haematoma) requires a relaxed pain-free patient so that the surgeon has the best conditions for what can be a difficult procedure. The relaxed pain-free perineum provided by a spinal or epidural anaesthetic gives excellent operating conditions for these procedures.

The block required for these procedures is primarily of the sacral roots (a saddle block), and a running epidural may be topped up using 10 ml of bupivacaine 0.5%.

The epidural or top-up is best given in the sitting position, but this may not be practical if the patient finds this to be uncomfortable due to the injured perineum. It is important that any hidden blood loss should be taken into consideration.

After the procedure, the epidural can continue to provide analgesia using a low concentration top-up or by means of epidural opiate, assuming that adequate nursing care is available.

If there is no epidural in place then spinal anaesthesia can be used to provide the sacral block, 1.5 ml heavy bupivacaine will be sufficient. It is important to remember that the woman may find the sitting position for insertion very uncomfortable and it is usually best to insert the block in the left lateral position.

9 Epidurals in labour for women with medical problems

Successive Confidential Enquiry into Maternal Deaths and Deaths in Infancy (CEMACH) reports have recommended the need for multidisciplinary team planning for women with concurrent medical disease. The initial booking history is important in ensuring that those women with medical problems have the appropriate advice and investigations in the antenatal period and are delivered in an appropriate environment. Women for example with complex cardiac disease will need input from cardiologists, obstetricians, anaesthetists and other health care professionals so that a considered plan is made for the management of the pregnancy and delivery. Women with less complex problems can essentially be treated as normal.

There is no place for women with complex medical problems to only first meet the anaesthetist when in labour. This chapter aims to clarify the problems of women with medical disease and the place of epidural analgesia for these women as well as the place of the anaesthetist within the team including their role in high dependency and intensive care.

The consideration of epidural analgesia in patients with medical diseases depends upon a basic understanding of the nature of the disease in question, together with an appreciation of the potential effects of an epidural on the disease. A possible interaction of the epidural with any medication that the patient may be taking should also be taken into account.

The following medical conditions are discussed in this chapter:

- cardiovascular disease
- respiratory disease
- endocrine disorders
- neurological disease
- renal disease
- heamatological disorders
- skeletal deformities
- obesity
- potential anaesthetic problems
- substance abuse
- the sick maternity patient – HDU and ITU care.

Cardiovascular disease

The most common cardiac problems presenting in pregnancy are congenital heart disease and rheumatic heart disease. Less commonly seen but currently on the increase are the cardiomyopathies and myocardial ischaemia.

Decisions about how to manage the cardiac patient during delivery should be made by the obstetrician and the anaesthetist before labour commences. To a large extent these decisions will be based on the severity of the heart disease. A rational method of grading such patients is provided by the New York Heart Association classification, which estimates cardiac disability from the patient's present and past disability.

Assessment of cardiac disability

Class 1: patients without limitation of physical activity. Ordinary physical activity does not cause undue fatigue, palpitations, dyspnoea or anginal pain.

Class 2: patients with slight limitation of physical activity. They are comfortable at rest but ordinary physical activity results in fatigue, palpitations, dyspnoea or anginal pain.

Class 3: patients with marked limitation of physical activity. They are comfortable at rest but less than ordinary physical activity causes fatigue, palpitations, dyspnoea or anginal pain.

Class 4: patients with inability to carry out any physical activity without discomfort. Symptoms of cardiac insufficiency or anginal syndrome may be present even at rest. If any physical activity is undertaken, discomfort is increased.

Patients in classes 3 and 4 are the main cause of concern to the anaesthetist.

In addition to the assessment of the degree of cardiac disability as described above, it is important to understand the effect of the usual stresses and physiological changes associated with childbirth on the disease process and also the effect that an epidural may have on the disease.

The stresses that are normally encountered in labour

1. First stage of labour: painful uterine contractions; work involved in uterine contractions.
2. Second stage of labour: painful contractions and the additional work of delivering the baby.
3. Third stage of labour: a major redistribution of blood in the cardiovascular system occurs during and after delivery of the placenta.

The effects of epidural analgesia on cardiac disease

The abolition of pain

Pain in labour increases blood pressure and pulse rate. Both can be deleterious to all classes of cardiac disability, but particularly to classes 3 and 4. Epidural analgesia is the most reliable method of producing a pain-free labour.

The sympathetic blockade

A full account of the mechanism of sympathetic blockade is given in Chapter 6. In brief, an epidural anaesthetic blocks the sympathetic nervous system as well as the sensory and motor nerve pathways. The effect of this is to produce a peripheral vasodilatation in the area of the blocked segments. In assessing the possible effects of this peripheral vasodilatation it is important first to decide the degree of strain on the right or left side of the heart.

Left heart failure would benefit from the degree of sympathetic vasodilatation produced by the epidural. This is due to the fact that vasodilatation reduces the resistance against which the heart has to pump so that the work of the heart is eased.

Right heart failure, particularly related to a heart defect that produces a left to right shunt, poses more serious problems as systemic blood pressure changes may lead to a reversal of the shunt and hence a more careful assessment is required.

When is it safe to perform an epidural in the presence of heart disease?

Arriving at a decision as to whether epidural analgesia would be advisable for a particular cardiac patient may be aided by the following guidelines.

1. In any disease with a degree of left ventricular failure epidural analgesia will be **beneficial** by reducing pain and by the vasodilatation effect described above.
2. In a heart condition where a drop in peripheral vascular resistance would be deleterious, for example where aortic stenosis, pulmonary hypertension and hypertrophic cardiomyopathy are present epidural analgesia may be contraindicated.

The place of epidural analgesia in patients with cardiac problems

Childbirth should be planned to produce the least disturbance of the cardiovascular system. Epidural analgesia has its place to play in achieving this in the following classes of cardiac disability.

Women with minimal cardiovascular impairment (classes 1 and 2)

Epidural analgesia should be offered as it will provide a less stressful labour than other methods of pain relief. The abolition of pain following a good epidural block prevents the reflex rise in blood pressure and increase in pulse rate associated with pain (see Chapter 6).

The management of the second stage of labour will depend upon the functional disability of the woman and whether she is fit enough to do the work involved in a normal second stage. Most women in this group will enjoy a normal second stage, but should help be required by assisted vaginal delivery then the epidural can be topped up accordingly.

Women with moderate cardiovascular impairment (class 3)

The aim of maintaining cardiovascular stability in this group is even more important. Therefore greater care and attention will be required whilst administering epidural analgesia in order to avoid pain with its associated rise in blood pressure and pulse rate and to minimize the vasodilatation effect of sympathetic blockade. There are two techniques that may help to achieve these aims.

1. The sympathetic blockade associated with epidural analgesia can be minimized by keeping the dose of local anaesthetic small and by giving it in divided doses or by low dose infusion (see Chapter 7).
2. Opiates (see Chapter 5) can be added to the local anaesthetic for the epidural. This allows less local anaesthetic to be used, which in turn minimizes the vasodilatation effect described above and so cardiovascular instability is reduced.

Women with severe cardiovascular impairment (class 4)

Patients in this group will be a challenge to both obstetric and anaesthetic staff. Their management requires intensive care and detailed monitoring.

Monitoring

Careful monitoring is advisable in the management of epidural analgesia for cardiac patients. It should include the following.

1. **Blood pressure:**
   (a) routine non-invasive blood pressure measurement by automatic monitor (for example 'Dinamap')
   (b) invasive blood pressure measurement (via an arterial line).
2. **Pulse rate:** if possible this should be measured by a continuous electrocardiographic monitor.

3. **Fluid balance:** intake and output measured by a fluid balance chart (catheterization will be necessary to measure urine output).
4. **Central venous pressure (CVP) monitoring:** a CVP catheter may be inserted via an arm vein (less commonly via the internal jugular vein – a more uncomfortable procedure for the patient) and sited in or nearer to the superior vena cava where it reflects the pressure in the right side of the heart. This pressure is an indicator of fluid overload or hypovolaemia.
5. **Swan Ganz catheter:** a Swan Ganz catheter is usually inserted via the internal jugular vein in the neck. It is a specialized device, which can be guided through the right side of the heart into the pulmonary vasculature. This enables the pulmonary wedge pressure (which reflects left heart pressure) and cardiac output to be monitored.

Monitors 1, 2 and 3 are routinely used in all classes of cardiac disability. Monitors 4 and 5 may be added when managing patients with class 3 and 4 disability levels.

All cardiac patients should be nursed in a single room with constant midwife supervision, preferably a midwife trained in high dependency care. The most severely ill will require full intensive care management. A careful record should be kept of all monitoring in addition to the usual partogram. A large high dependency chart is useful for this purpose and may prevent any possible confusion arising from using several smaller charts.

Caesarean section in cardiac patients

In those patients where it has been decided that the best means of delivery is by Caesarean section the anaesthetist is faced with the decision as to which is the safer form of anaesthetic – general or regional.

As long as the patient's cardiac condition is compatible the author's preference is for a combined spinal epidural or epidural anaesthesia, but each anaesthetist will perform best the technique he or she is most used to. As this is not the occasion for experimentation, for many anaesthetists the safest technique would undoubtedly be a general anaesthetic.

Interaction of epidural analgesia with medication in heart disease

Many cardiac patients, particularly those in classes 3 and 4, may be on medication for their condition. Any possible interaction between such treatment and the epidural should be considered. The drugs most commonly seen are the following:

1. anticoagulants
2. digoxin

3. diuretics
4. beta-blockers.

Anticoagulants

Epidural analgesia is **contraindicated** if the patient is anticoagulated. This would most commonly be encountered in patients who have had a heart valve replacement or who are in atrial fibrillation.

However, in specific instances where the benefits afforded by epidural analgesia are thought to be important in the management of labour, the anticoagulant may be stopped before the delivery so that the epidural may be sited and removed whilst the patient's clotting screen is normal.

Digoxin

There are no interactions between digoxin and an epidural. Any effects should be beneficial where digoxin slows the heart rate (for example atrial fibrillation) to a more normal rate.

Diuretics

The prolonged use of diuretics may predispose the patient to dehydration. Therefore care will be needed with fluid balance in order to maintain systolic blood pressure when the sympathetic blockade effect of the epidural produces vasodilatation.

Beta-blockers

Beta-blockers are used in the treatment of angina and cardiomyopathies with or without hypertension. The effect of particular relevance to epidural analgesia is that the patient's heart rate may not increase in response to a drop in blood pressure. Such a drop may occur as a result of the sympathetic blockade as mentioned above or as a result of hypovolaemia.

Cardiac arrhythmias

These should be evaluated as in non-pregnant patients, and any underlying cardiac lesion investigated and appropriately treated. Benign arrhythmias and palpitations are common in pregnancy and may be asymptomatic.

Cardiac arrhythmias in themselves are not a contraindication to epidural analgesia provided that any underlying cardiac lesion or treatment is taken into account.

Hypertension

Essential hypertension may coexist with pregnancy and may be exacerbated by pre-eclampsia. Epidural analgesia is an integral part of the management of patients with hypertension in labour, whatever the cause. Care must be taken if the patient is already on antihypertensive therapy as this may act synergistically with the sympathetic block of the epidural. Stress should be kept to a minimum in these women and pain relief must be effective.

It should be remembered that hypertension may be associated with underlying pathology, for example coronary artery insufficiency and renal disease.

Respiratory disease

The most common pulmonary disease encountered in pregnant women is asthma. Bronchiectasis and cystic fibrosis are less common.

Asthma

Many women suffering from asthma are troubled less with this complaint during pregnancy than at other times. A few find that their asthma is much worse.

Some of the factors that can exacerbate an asthmatic attack, for example anxiety, pain and hyperventilation, are found in childbirth. Epidural analgesia is recommended in asthmatics in order to achieve the following:

- stress-free labour
- pain-free labour
- no hyperventilation
- a fully awake patient able to use inhalers as required.

Administering a general anaesthetic to an asthmatic may be a hazardous procedure. A good epidural sited in good time should avoid the need for general anaesthesia should Caesarean section become necessary.

Bronchiectasis and cystic fibrosis

The main problem in patients suffering from bronchiectasis and cystic fibrosis is that secretions are continually produced from the diseased area of their lungs. These secretions must be removed by regular postural drainage to prevent their accumulation in the lungs and an ensuing chest infection. Patients with these conditions are also prone to shortness of breath on exertion and attacks of wheezing.

Epidural analgesia is recommended for the same reasons given above for asthma, with the added benefit that the patient is able to continue with regular postural drainage more easily throughout labour.

It is particularly important to avoid a general anaesthetic in these patients because of the risk of anaesthetic problems and post-operative chest infections. Therefore an epidural given in early labour may be topped up to provide epidural analgesia in the event that Caesarean section may become necessary.

Endocrine disorders

The endocrine disorders commonly encountered in pregnancy are:

- diabetes
- thyroid disorders
- diseases of the adrenal cortex
  - Addison's disease
  - Cushing's syndrome
  - Conn's syndrome.

Diabetes

Diabetes is the most common endocrine disorder seen in women of child-bearing age. The diabetes may be gestational (occurring during pregnancy) or non-gestational (present before pregnancy). The patients most likely to have problems with control of blood sugar during labour and delivery are those who are insulin dependent at the time of the delivery.

In labour such a diabetic will not be taking food and so she will require a regime of insulin and dextrose to control her blood sugar. Usually the insulin will be given intravenously by a syringe pump. Careful monitoring will avoid hypoglycaemia or ketoacidosis, both of which may cause problems for mother and baby.

Epidural analgesia is recommended for these patients as the abolition of pain and stress will contribute to better control of blood glucose. Pain and anxiety reflexly stimulate the adrenal gland to secrete adrenaline, nor-adrenaline and cortisol into the circulation. These substances in turn increase blood sugar levels, making the control of diabetes in labour more difficult. Epidural analgesia significantly reduces this effect. A full description of these physiological changes is given in Chapter 6.

Diabetes and Caesarean section

Many insulin-dependent diabetic patients are likely to require Caesarean section either electively or during labour. This is due to the fact that diabetes is associated with poor placental function and macrosomia.

Epidural anaesthesia is advised as it will cause less disturbance to blood sugar levels than a general anaesthetic. This is due to the fact that epidural analgesia blocks the nerve impulses from the operation site, thus reducing the stress response (described above) that these impulses would have produced.

Thyroid disorders

Thyrotoxicosis is the most common thyroid problem seen in young child-bearing women. Myxoedema is rarely encountered in this age group.

Most patients embarking on pregnancy with pre-existing thyrotoxicosis are well controlled on an appropriate dose of carbimazole (they probably would not have conceived if they were not). However, the activity of the thyroid gland will increase during pregnancy, and if the dose of carbimazole has not been adjusted the patient may present in labour with mild to moderate symptoms of thyrotoxicosis. In markedly thyrotoxic patients epidural analgesia can help prevent a thyroid crisis – an emergency caused by uncontrolled outpouring of thyroid hormones into the circulation.

Diseases of the adrenal cortex

The adrenal cortex secretes the hormones cortisol and aldosterone. When dysfunction occurs there may be underproduction of these hormones (Addison's disease) or overproduction of cortisol (Cushing's syndrome) or aldosterone (Conn's syndrome).

The relevance of these rare diseases to epidural analgesia is that the adrenocortical hormones are normally produced in response to pain and stress, both of which occur in labour. Insufficient hormone production results in an abnormal stress response; over-production results in secondary diseases.

Addison's disease

Patients who suffer from Addison's disease do not produce sufficient adrenocortical hormones and their treatment consists of a maintenance dose of fludrocortisone and hydrocortisone. They are unable to respond to stressful situations, such as labour, with an automatic increase in the levels of these hormones as occurs in the normal patient. There are many possible consequences of this, of which the most serious is a sudden profound drop in blood pressure.

Epidural analgesia commenced early in the labour of a patient with Addison's disease can abolish pain, anxiety and stress, thus minimizing this complication.

Cushing's syndrome

Cushing's syndrome is usually caused by a pituitary adenoma, which secretes excessive amounts of adrenocorticotrophic hormone (ACTH). This in turn causes the adrenal cortex to produce large amounts of cortisol. The secondary effects of overproduction of cortisol relevant to epidural analgesia are as follows:

- obesity
- hypertension
- diabetes.

Each of these conditions (discussed in separate sections in this book) may themselves be an indication for an epidural.

The features of Cushing's syndrome may also be seen where there has been prolonged treatment by corticosteroids for other medical conditions.

Neurological disease

There is a degree of resistance and anxiety concerning the use of epidural analgesia and anaesthesia in patients with neurological disease. However, in most instances, after logical consideration of the problem, an epidural will prove to be the analgesic of choice in the management of labour in this group of patients. It is important that the anaesthetist understands each disease and is able to discuss with the patient any risk factors or particular problems pertaining to the use of an epidural in the presence of that disease.

Patients may present in pregnancy suffering from one of a variety of neurological diseases. Whilst none of these are seen very frequently, those most commonly encountered in the childbearing age group are described below and the place epidural analgesia has to play is given below.

Spina bifida

There are two types of spina bifida: spina bifida occulta and true spina bifida.

Spina bifida occulta

This condition is usually asymptomatic and undiagnosed, and may be discovered coincidentally either by the presence of a hairy dimple in the midline of the lumbar or sacral area of the patient's back or by the palpation of a bifid spinous process in the same area.

Either of these signs may be noticed only after positioning a patient prior to inserting an epidural. If the epidural is sited at or near the level of spina bifida occulta there is a slightly greater chance of dural puncture owing to possible minor variations in the anatomy external to the epidural space. This risk should be explained to the patient. The risk of dural puncture lessens the further away from the affected spinous process the epidural is sited.

Spina bifida cystica

Spina bifida cystica is defined as incomplete closure of the spinal canal. Those defects compatible with survival are surgically repaired in the neonatal period, and the resulting neurological deficit can vary from severe paralysis of the lower limbs with bladder and bowel dysfunction to practically no discernible problems. This condition is associated with the spinal cord terminating at a low level and tethering of the spinal cord. Caution must be used when inserting a regional block and as low a level as possible should be used for spinal anaesthesia.

The presence of spina bifida (regardless of the degree of neurological deficit) is not a contraindication to an epidural, as the site of surgical repair is usually below the level at which the epidural would be placed. Any impairment of function present before the epidural will not be adversely affected by the epidural. The local anaesthetic may not spread well into the area of the spina bifida and though good first-stage analgesia is usually achieved the sacral roots may be spared therefore the block does not work so well for second-stage or may not top up well for a Caesarean section.

However, as for spina bifida occulta, there is a slightly increased risk of dural puncture and the patient should be informed of this risk before proceeding with the epidural.

Cerebral tumours

An epidural can be given in the presence of a cerebral tumour provided that the intracranial pressure is not raised.

If the intracranial pressure is raised, an inadvertent dural puncture whilst siting the epidural may cause sudden lowering of pressure in the CSF in the spinal canal. This in turn may cause coning of the medulla at the foramen ovale owing to the pressure difference between the CSF surrounding the brain and the CSF surrounding the spinal cord with catastrophic consequences.

There may be instances where a painful stressful labour in a patient with a cerebral tumour causing raised intracranial pressure may be dangerous (e.g. where there is a risk of haemorrhage into the tumour). In such a case the benefits of an epidural may outweigh the risk of a dural puncture. Such a procedure should only be carried out by an experienced obstetric anaesthetist.

Cerebrovascular accidents

This group includes cerebral aneurysms (pre- and post-surgical repair), cerebral haemorrhage and cerebral thrombosis. Some of the women who have had a cerebral thrombosis may have a thrombophilia and be on prophylactic low molecular weight heparin (see below).

Epidural analgesia is not contraindicated in patients suffering from any of these conditions. Indeed, a pain-free and stress-free labour provided by an epidural may be an advantage as pain and stress may cause a rise in blood pressure and intracranial pressure, which could adversely affect any of these conditions.

Degenerative neurological diseases

Multiple sclerosis

Multiple sclerosis is a disease of unknown aetiology characterized clinically by symptoms that indicate the presence of multiple lesions in the white matter of the brain and spinal cord. The disease runs a relapsing and remitting course, usually over many years, resulting in progressive paralysis and lack of coordination.

Epidural analgesia is recommended in women suffering from multiple sclerosis as it is possible that any symptoms present during pregnancy may be exacerbated by a painful and stressful labour. Also, as muscle power is often reduced and coordination impaired, a normal delivery may be impossible. In anticipation of this an epidural will allow a pain-free assisted vaginal delivery. However, owing to the naturally relapsing and remitting course of the disease the anaesthetist may feel reticent to perform an epidural, fearing that a chance relapse in the puerperium would be blamed on the epidural.

Therefore it is important that such patients and their partners should be seen by the anaesthetist during the antenatal period so that analgesia in labour can be discussed and planned.

Friedreich's ataxia

Friedreich's ataxia is the most common of a group of degenerative hereditary ataxias characterized by spastic paraplegia, cerebellar ataxia and impaired positional sensation. Scoliosis and myocardial degeneration may be additional features.

Epidural analgesia in labour is recommended for the same reasons as in multiple sclerosis, as is antenatal counselling by the anaesthetist. The possibility of associated scoliosis and myocardial degeneration call for a careful antenatal anaesthetic assessment.

Post-infective problems

Poliomyelitis

Poliomyelitis is a virus infection, which may cause damage to the brain and spinal cord, producing varying degrees of paralysis. There is no contraindication to epidural analgesia in patients who have suffered from poliomyelitis, but technical difficulties should be anticipated where there are associated skeletal abnormalities or respiratory difficulties.

Meningitis

The main problem concerning epidural analgesia in women who have a past history of viral or bacterial meningitis is that the disease may have caused scarring of the meninges, which may result in obliteration of the epidural space. This is more common after bacterial meningitis. The effect of this is to increase the risk of dural puncture whilst performing an epidural. This risk must be balanced against the strength of the indication for an epidural in each patient.

Post-infective neuropathy

Conditions such as Guillain-Barré usually leave no permanent neurological disability though the woman is often left with a fear of being paralysed and a fear of lumbar puncture. It is important that these women are seen antenatally and are reassured about regional block for childbirth and will be treated sympathetically by the obstetric anaesthetist.

Myalgic encephalitis or post-viral fatigue syndrome

Myalgic encephalitis is believed to be a post-viral condition, but the aetiology is not proven and its very existence is disputed by some. Whatever the cause, it is presenting in an increasing number of pregnant women. They may have varying degrees of disability, but a common factor is that they are easily fatigued by exertion. They may also have a low pain threshold. Therefore the desirability of a pain-free and stress-free labour in these patients is a strong recommendation for epidural analgesia.

Myasthenia gravis

Myasthenia gravis is a disease of the neuromuscular junction associated with an abnormal degree of fatiguability of skeletal muscle. The disease is controlled by a combination of anticholinergic drugs (for example neostigmine or pyridostigmine) and vagolitic drugs (for example atropine or propantheline); the latter are used to counteract the side-effects of the former.

Epidural analgesia is recommended in patients suffering from myasthenia gravis for the following reasons:

- to allow oral medication to be continued throughout labour (in the absence of pain in labour gastric emptying is not significantly affected)
- to reduce the work that they have to do in labour (their muscles may not be capable of sustaining the normal effort of labour)
- to reduce hyperventilation in response to pain, thus preventing undue fatigue of their respiratory muscles
- in anticipation of an instrumental delivery

- to avoid a general anaesthetic should Caesarean section become necessary (patients with myasthenia gravis have an increased sensitivity to muscle relaxants, which, when given with a general anaesthetic, can lead to the necessity of post-operative ventilation).

Epilepsy

Epilepsy is a transient disorder of consciousness often associated with sensory or motor phenomena, and it is treated with a variety of anticonvulsant drugs. An epileptic attack may be triggered by many circumstances, including pain, stress and fatigue in labour. Therefore epidural analgesia is recommended in labour in order to minimize the possibility of triggering an epileptic attack.

However, it should be borne in mind that the local anaesthetic agents used in epidural analgesia may themselves have convulsive properties (see Chapter 5) and so the safe maximum dose may be significantly lower.

Renal disease

Patients suffering from renal disease present in three broad categories.

1. Pre-existing renal disease: the illness may be exacerbated by the demands of pregnancy.
2. Renal disease acquired as a result of a pregnancy complication, for example pre-eclampsia.
3. Post-renal transplant: renal function may be normal in these cases but they may be on a complicated drug regime.

Epidurals and renal disease

Patients suffering from renal disease may be debilitated from one or more effects of the condition:

- electrolyte disturbance
- anaemia
- hypertension
- drugs, for example antihypertensives, diuretics.

Epidural analgesia is recommended in labour as all the above problems may be adversely affected by stress. In post-renal transplant patients stress could initiate a rejection of the transplant.

An epidural anaesthetic is also recommended as a general anaesthetic may be contraindicated, particularly if there is electrolyte imbalance (a raised serum potassium may be further elevated by the effect of a depolarizing muscle relaxant). Particular note should be made of any item of the patient's medication that may interact with the effect of the local anaesthetic used in the epidural, for example beta-blockers and diuretics, which are discussed above.

Owing to the complex nature of renal problems, a nephrologist's opinion should be sought (if one is not already involved) early in the antenatal period.

Haematological disorders

Patients who may bleed

The place of epidural analgesia must be carefully considered where anticoagulation or a bleeding disorder coexists. The majority of maternity patients who may bleed excessively fall into the following groups:

1. those who are fully anticoagulated with heparin or warfarin
2. those who are receiving heparin or low molecular weight heparin
3. those who are taking anti-platelet agents
4. those who are suffering from thrombocytopenia.

Patients who are fully anticoagulated with heparin or warfarin

Epidural analgesia is contraindicated in the presence of full anticoagulation with heparin or warfarin. If there is a strong indication for an epidural, the anticoagulant should be stopped or the dose reduced and the epidural inserted when the clotting time has returned to normal, provided that this is compatible with the medical reasons for anticoagulation.

Patients receiving subcutaneous heparin

There are two groups of patients who are receiving subcutaneous heparin, usually in the form of low molecular weight heparin:

- women with previous history of deep vein thrombosis (DVT) or pulmonary embolus (PE)
- women with a known thrombophilia.

Women with previous history of DVT or PE are usually on a prophylactic dose of low molecular weight heparin (LMWH) and the insertion or removal of an epidural catheter should be avoided for 12 hours after the administration of the low molecular weight heparin.

Women with a known thrombophilia are hypercoagulable when untreated with anticoagulants and the anaesthetist should be able to assess the risks and benefits of a regional block in this group of patients. The timing of the insertion of a regional block may need to be a consultant decision and if this is so then this must be clearly stated in the medical record.

Generally all patients on LMWH should be advised to omit an imminent dose of LMWH if they think they are in labour and to come into hospital.

During labour these women should be kept well hydrated and as mobile as possible.

Those women who are on heparin should not have an epidural catheter inserted or removed for 1–2 hours after the dose of heparin.

A plan should be made in the antenatal period for the management of these women and the risks and benefits of regional block should have been discussed with the woman.

Patients suffering from thrombocytopenia

Thrombocytopenia may be associated with pre-eclampsia. In this case it would be considered safe to proceed with an epidural where the platelet count is above 100 000. Below this count the decision to proceed would depend on the results of a clotting screen.

In cases where there are other causes for the thrombocytopenia, it would be safe to offer an epidural if the platelet count is above 50 000 if the clotting screen results are acceptable.

In both instances the advice of a haematologist may be helpful.

Haemoglobinopathies

Many types of haemoglobinopathy exist, but the one of clinical significance is the haemoglobin variant HbS, a hereditary condition found in African and Mediterranean peoples.

This haemoglobin predisposes to a 'sickling' distortion of red blood cells at low oxygen saturation (see below). The result is that the red blood cells block the capillaries instead of flowing through them. Sickle cells have a shorter life and this predisposes to anaemia.

Heterozygotic patients (that is patients with 'sickle-cell trait') should pose no problems in pregnancy although situations that could produce a low oxygen saturation (e.g. problems during a general anaesthetic) should be avoided.

Homozygotic patients are often severely ill in pregnancy due to anaemia. Meticulous care is required to avoid situations that may exacerbate 'sickling' of the red blood cells in the capillaries, which can cause tissue infarction and ischaemic pain. In labour such a problem may arise due to:

- hypoxia
- dehydration
- hypotension (including aorto-caval compression)
- acidosis.

Epidural analgesia is indicated as the reduction of pain and stress will help prevent these problems from developing. However, extra care should be taken in its administration, particularly to minimize hypotension and aorto-caval compression. Therefore careful monitoring, including oxygen saturation, is recommended. In severe cases continuous oxygen administration is often necessary.

Thalassaemias

Thalassaemia is an inherited disease, which results in defective haemoglobin synthesis. The condition produces anaemia of varying degrees from very mild to fatally severe (thalassaemia minor, thalassaemia intermedia and thalassaemia major). The indication for an epidural depends upon the degree of anaemia.

Skeletal deformities

Skeletal deformities can cause technical difficulties with intubation for general anaesthesia or cause technical difficulties with inserting an epidural.

Deformities that make epidural insertion difficult

- Spina bifida (discussed above)
- Scoliosis (including those women who have had surgery)
- Chronic back problems (for example prolapsed intervertebral disc)
- Previous surgical intervention (for example laminectomy).

None of these conditions is a contraindication to epidural analgesia, although their presence may cause the insertion of the epidural to be more difficult.

Patients who suffer from chronic back problems (particularly those with disc lesions) should be reassured that the insertion of an epidural will not damage their back nor will it worsen their existing back problem. A useful point to make is that epidural analgesia is extensively used in the treatment of a variety of back problems. Time taken to explain where the epidural space is in relation to the intervertebral disc will also help to allay anxiety.

All patients with back problems should be nursed carefully in labour (with or without epidural) so that the lumbar spine is maintained in a good position.

Obesity

The obese woman presents many problems to the anaesthetist and the obstetric team throughout pregnancy and labour. General anaesthesia in particular carries significant risks.

Problems created by obesity in pregnancy and labour

- An increased incidence of diabetes
- An increased incidence of hypertension
- A larger volume of acidic gastric contents and increased incidence of hiatus hernia
- A greater risk of aorto-caval compression
- Difficulty in monitoring the baby
- Increased risk of DVT
- Increased risk of wound infection.

Problems created by obesity with general anaesthesia

- Venepuncture may be difficult.
- Positioning on the operating table can be difficult.
- There is an increased risk of aorto-caval compression.
- Ventilation may be difficult. Decreased vital capacity and functional residual volume together with splinting of the diaphragm can cause underventilation of the dependent areas of the lung with a risk of hypoxia. Many of these women desaturate when laid flat.
- Intubation may be difficult. Obesity is often accompanied by large breasts, which obstruct the laryngoscope handle. Pre-eclampsia can exaggerate the oedema of the upper airways and mouth associated with pregnancy.
- Surgery is technically more difficult. Obese patients may also suffer a greater than average blood loss during surgery.

Epidural analgesia and obesity

The above points illustrate the potential problems produced by obesity in pregnancy and labour. Many of these problems can be helped by an epidural, particularly the avoidance of the hazards of a general anaesthetic.

However, the insertion of an epidural in an obese patient can itself be difficult and is often a challenge to even the most experienced anaesthetist. A further problem is that once effective, any loss of movement in the patient's legs caused by the epidural may cause nursing problems.

Performing an epidural in the obese patient

Detecting the epidural space is difficult as each of the ligamentous layers encountered by the epidural needle are infiltrated by fatty tissue. The effect of this is that the ligaments feel soft and less well defined. Therefore it becomes more difficult to detect a positive loss of resistance as the epidural needle penetrates the ligamentum flavum. The use of ultrasound for these women has been discussed in Chapter 3.

Potential anaesthetic problems

- Skeletal deformities
- Suxamethonium sensitivity
- Allergies (drugs and latex).

Deformities that make intubation for general anaesthesia difficult

- Small underslung jaw
- Immobile neck
- Small mouth opening (for example caused by scleroderma).

Intubation in pregnancy can itself be a difficult procedure. An anaesthetist's nightmare would be to meet any of the above problems for the first time at emergency Caesarean section. It is far more preferable to have the problem identified at antenatal assessment or early in labour, perhaps having been alerted by a past history of difficult or failed intubation. In some cases the past history may be the only clue where otherwise the patient appears perfectly normal.

This problem is an indication for an epidural to be sited early in labour. This may then be topped up as required for operative delivery or Caesarean section.

Suxamethonium sensitivity

Suxamethonium sensitivity is a strong indication for epidural anaesthesia. Suxamethonium is a depolarizing muscle relaxant used mainly to facilitate intubation in the rapid sequence induction of general anaesthesia, for example for Caesarean section.

Suxamethonium sensitivity occurs when there is a deficiency of the enzyme plasma cholinesterase, which is normally present in the body in sufficient quantity to metabolize and so reverse the effects of suxamethonium within 5–10 minutes of its administration. The effect of suxamethonium sensitivity is that the drug will last longer in the circulation than normally – as long as 24 hours where there is complete absence of plasma cholinesterase – and the patient will require ventilatory support throughout this period. Therefore a general anaesthetic should be avoided if possible.

Allergies (drugs and latex)

A careful history of the allergy and its significance should be taken in the antenatal period allowing time to retrieve old medical records and seek the help of the immunologist and pharmacist where appropriate. Where a true allergy is identified the records should be clearly annotated and where relevant the patient advised to carry an Epipen (a pre-filled syringe containing a measured dose of adrenaline) and wear a Medialert tag.

Women who have had a bad experience with opiates or general anaesthesia are often worried about the choice of pain relief in labour and epidural analgesia may be the pain relief option of choice for these women.

Those women with latex allergy can be divided into those with a mild skin reaction on contact with latex and those with a major life threatening anaphylaxis on the smallest contact with latex. All these women can be reassured that epidural analgesia is safe and that anaesthetic equipment is latex free. All units should have a latex allergy guideline and latex-free equipment should be available preferably on a special trolley for those women with severe problems.

Substance abuse

Drug abuse in the general population is sufficiently prevalent to be considered a potential complication in the management of labour. Drug abuse is too easily overlooked, and often diagnosis depends upon the anaesthetist's first having considered the possibility.

The drugs most commonly abused are as follows:

1. nicotine
2. alcohol
3. opiates
4. marijuana
5. cocaine.

Nicotine

Nicotine is undoubtedly the most common addictive drug taken regularly by a significant number of pregnant women. The medical problems associated with regular smoking are well known:

- chest problems (for example bronchitis)
- chest problems associated with general anaesthesia (for example bronchospasm, hypoxia)
- stimulation of the autonomic ganglia with peripheral vasoconstriction and hypertension

- association with a fetus that is small for gestational age
- placental abruption.

Epidural analgesia should be encouraged in heavy smokers to avoid the risks ensuing from general anaesthesia with these patients such as bronchoconstriction and hypoxia during anaesthesia, and hypoxia and chest infections post-operatively.

Alcohol

Alcohol usually only causes problems in maternity patients when heavy drinking has occurred throughout pregnancy. Such patients may need careful counselling and management, and potential medical problems associated with high alcohol consumption should be excluded:

- fetal alcohol syndrome
- maternal problems (anaemia, cardiomyopathy, liver disease, peripheral neuropathy).

Pain in labour is best managed by epidural analgesia to avoid interactions between pethidine and alcohol, but the increased risks of an epidural in patients who have the above medical complications of alcohol abuse must be taken into account.

Opiate addiction

The most common form of opiate to be abused is heroin. Pain relief in labour and general anaesthesia, if required, can be a problem with heroin addicts owing to tolerance to opiates. Many of these women manage to get off the heroin and are on a maintenance dose of methadone, which must be continued throughout labour and delivery. Epidural analgesia and anaesthesia is the obvious way of avoiding problems, but associated conditions should be taken into consideration:

- difficult intravenous access
- association with hepatitis and AIDS
- poor nutrition with the possibility of anaemia.

Marijuana

Marijuana is usually taken as a recreational drug rather than as a drug of addiction. As a beta-adrenergic agonist it can affect the circulation:

- increased blood pressure
- increased pulse rate
- increase in the workload of the heart.

An additional effect is that smoking marijuana increases carbon monoxide levels in the lungs to a greater extent than with cigarette smoking, and this may cause respiratory problems if general anaesthesia is administered. It should also be remembered that marijuana abuse is often associated with tobacco and alcohol abuse.

For these reasons epidural analgesia and anaesthesia are preferred, but careful monitoring of the cardiovascular system is recommended. If the patient is acutely intoxicated, sedation may first be helpful, for example with a benzodiazepine.

Cocaine

Cocaine can be taken as snuff or smoked in the form of the alkaloid 'crack'. The abuse of cocaine can cause problems in pregnancy and during labour owing to its stimulant effect on the central nervous and cardiovascular systems resulting from the blocking of the pre-synaptic uptake of nora-drenaline, serotonin and dopamine. These effects may cause an increase in blood pressure, heart rate and peripheral resistance, and may present as follows:

- placental abruption
- cerebral haemorrhage
- hallucinations
- myocardial ischaemia.

Cocaine also has local anaesthetic effects and can lower the seizure threshold. The effects of raised blood pressure may be mistaken for pre-eclampsia.

Labour is best managed by epidural analgesia with careful monitoring of the cardiovascular system.

The sick maternity patient – HDU and ITU care

Some of these women particularly those with cardiac disease will be sick and require multidisciplinary care and high dependency or intensive care. Whether this is provided on the delivery suite or not depends on the severity of the disease and the availability of suitably trained staff of all disciplines to care for the woman.

10 Problems associated with epidurals

Introduction

As a general rule any medical procedure or administration of a drug, no matter how 'safe' it is thought to be, can cause problems or produce complications or side-effects. Epidural analgesia is no exception to this rule. Therefore epidural analgesia should always be performed with meticulous care to ensure the highest degree of safety.

In this chapter the main problems that may be encountered with epidural analgesia in both the intrapartum and postpartum periods are discussed. The effect of these problems can usually be minimized by early diagnosis and treatment.

As any problems that do arise may have medico-legal importance, three simple rules are of paramount importance:

1. full documentation of the problem as soon as is practicable
2. full explanation of the problem to the woman and her partner
3. consultant involvement for advice and support.

As described in Chapter 3 each stage in inserting the epidural catheter should be checked to ensure that the catheter is correctly placed. However, errors can be made and unforeseen problems can occur. It is important that the anaesthetist is continually vigilant so that such errors and problems can be promptly diagnosed and treated before serious consequences develop. The most effective way of dealing with a problem is to be equipped with a full understanding of the underlying cause.

Problems occurring during insertion of the epidural

Pain or paraesthesia during insertion of the catheter

A mild sensation of 'pins and needles' is commonly experienced during insertion of the epidural catheter. If pain or genuine paraesthesia occurs (particularly if localized to a nerve root) the attempt should be abandoned. The catheter should be withdrawn immediately (complete with the epidural needle) as injection of local anaesthetic solution directly into the nerve root can be injurious. A note should be made in the patient's records if pain or paraesthesia occurs on insertion of the catheter.

Vessel puncture

Management of the problem of blood in the epidural catheter is fully described in Chapter 3. The anaesthetist may continue with caution in the presence of a small amount of blood in the epidural catheter when the blood flushes away easily with saline. If it is clear that an epidural vein has been cannulated accidentally, the catheter (together with epidural needle) should be withdrawn to avoid the potentially serious consequences of intravenous injection of anaesthetic solution. In cases where doubt exists as to whether an epidural vein has been cannulated it is always safer to abandon the attempt and start again. All attempts should be fully documented.

Dural puncture

This is dealt with in Chapter 11.

Shearing of the epidural catheter

Shearing of the epidural catheter should not occur if one simple rule is adhered to: **never withdraw a catheter back through an epidural needle**. Any attempt to withdraw the catheter may damage, cut or shear it. A sheared catheter may not be noticed until it is removed from the patient when inspection reveals that it is incomplete. When this occurs, the removed portion of the catheter should be carefully packaged and attached to the patient's records. The portion of catheter that remains in the patient is inert and sterile and is unlikely to cause problems. Therefore it should be left undisturbed. The patient should be fully informed and reassured about this fact and a clear account of the episode should be made in the patient's records for future reference.

Fracture of the epidural needle

Fortunately, fracture of the epidural needle is a very rare occurrence. When it does happen the breakage is at the level of the wings or hub of the needle. Immediately this happens it is imperative to withdraw the remainder of the needle. An artery clip attached to the protruding broken needle end can be helpful. If the needle fracture is very near or just below the patient's skin retrieval can be difficult. In such instances urgent surgical removal of the needle is mandatory. In all cases the needle fracture should be fully reported to the manufacturer.

Problems occurring during epidural analgesia

Unilateral block

A true unilateral block is unusual – a block favouring one side of the body is more common. The most likely cause is that the epidural catheter has passed laterally, perhaps as far as the paravertebral space.

The more common occurrence of a block favouring one side can be managed as follows:

1. Position the patient with her unaffected side down and give a further dose of local anaesthetic (for example about half a top-up dose).
2. If there is no improvement, withdraw the catheter 1 cm and give another small top-up.

If this technique does not resolve the problem, the epidural should be resited. If the resited epidural still produces a true unilateral block, the presence of a mid-line fold in the epidural space may be suspected (see Chapter 2). The epidural should be abandoned and other analgesia offered.

Patchy block

A patchy block can occur when the top-up dose has been given too fast and/or during a uterine contraction. It usually resolves itself without treatment after the next top-up.

Persistent problems with a patchy block suggest that the epidural catheter is not well placed and should be replaced. If replacing the catheter does not resolve the problem, the possibility of fibrous bands in the epidural space preventing even spread of the local anaesthetic should be considered.

Missed segment

This can only be differentiated from an uneven block by careful sensory testing with a cold stimulus. The most commonly missed nerve root is L1, although why this should be so is unclear. A missed segment tends to occur at one top-up only and does not usually recur.

A missed segment is managed as follows:

1. Position the patient with the side of the unblocked segment down.
2. Give a top-up of 10–15 ml of bupivacaine 0.1% with 2 μg/ml fentanyl.
3. If this fails a top-up dose of 5 ml of bupivacaine 0.25% may be considered.

Groin pain

The first and most obvious reason to be excluded or dealt with is a full bladder. If groin pain persists and if it is associated with contractions, a vaginal examination will exclude full dilatation of the cervix. The obstetrician should be called if groin pain is present with a history of a scarred uterus. Groin pain as a symptom of impending dehiscence of a uterine scar is usually continuous and will break through an otherwise sound epidural block. It precedes more worrying signs such as changes in blood pressure, pulse rate and maternal or fetal distress.

Groin pain is usually due to a segmental nerve that has missed the effects of local anaesthetic – a missed segment.

Perineal pain

Perineal pain is usually associated with an occipito-posterior position of the baby's head, although it may also occur in a normal presentation. It can be treated by giving a top-up 10–15 ml of bupivacaine 0.1% with 2 µg/ml of fentanyl in the sitting position, which will extend the epidural block to include the sacral roots.

If this procedure fails to relieve the pain, the anaesthetist may consider giving fentanyl 25 µg diluted in saline via the epidural catheter.

Shivering

Shivering is a common occurrence during the course of an otherwise normal epidural. Although there are several theories, no single reason for this phenomenon has been identified. The most popular theory is that shivering is related to the temperature of the local anaesthetic solution. The presence of shivering is a nuisance, but it is not harmful to the patient unless it becomes so pronounced that it increases her oxygen requirements to the extent that she and the fetus may become hypoxic.

Hypotension

Supine hypotension is the most common cause of a fall in blood pressure in labour. It is caused by pressure of the gravid uterus on the aorta and inferior vena cava in a supine unwedged patient, and is fully discussed earlier in this chapter and in Chapter 6.

Any patient who is hypovolaemic due to dehydration or other cause of a low circulating blood volume (for example blood loss, pre-eclampsia) will have an exaggerated hypotensive response to the sympathetic block produced by the epidural. This should be corrected by the intravenous administration of crystalloid or colloid solutions or blood, whichever is clinically appropriate.

Hypotension due to an extensive epidural block is usually associated with an extensive sympathetic block. Corrective measures are as follows:

1. Check that the patient is in full lateral tilt.
2. Increase intravenous fluids – consider giving 500 ml of colloid quickly.
3. Give oxygen by face-mask.
4. If blood pressure remains low, give ephedrine intravenously in 3 mg boluses until a normal blood pressure is attained.

An accidental intrathecal injection should be suspected when a rapid fall in blood pressure occurs after a top-up – always first excluding supine hypotension.

Excessively high block

This is a profound and extensive block – sensory, motor and sympathetic – of the nervous system brought about by the effect of local anaesthetic solution on the spinal cord and spinal nerves. It can occur either when too much local anaesthetic is injected into the epidural space or when the local anaesthetic is injected into the wrong place. The diagnosis of the cause rests on the rate of onset and severity of symptoms. Some degree of hypotension is inevitable, respiratory and cardiovascular collapse may also occur.

Too much local anaesthetic (too large a volume or concentration)
This results in too great a spread of local anaesthetic in the epidural space. Reaction occurs 10–20 minutes after the event. The usual cause is that not enough care has been taken when topping up the epidural.

Injection of local anaesthetic into the wrong place
This occurs when the epidural catheter has been accidentally sited in the wrong place, resulting in either a subdural or intrathecal (spinal) injection of local anaesthetic.

With a subdural injection of local anaesthetic the reaction occurs 10–20 minutes after the injection. With a intrathecal (spinal) injection of local anaesthetic the reaction occurs within minutes.

In the event of an accidental massive spinal injection, the local anaesthetic rapidly reaches the medulla oblongata (the brainstem), causing **cardiorespiratory arrest**. Full facilities for rapid resuscitation should always be readily available when performing or topping up an epidural.

Convulsions are not usually part of the clinical picture as is the case when intravenous injection of local anaesthetic has occurred (see below).

Management of excessively high block

1. Call for help.
2. Initial 'ABC' (airway, breathing, circulation).
3. Give oxygen via a face-mask.
4. Tilt the patient laterally.
5. Give intravenous fluids.
6. Give ephedrine (3 mg intravenously, repeated as required).
   If required:
7. Maintain an airway – progressing from face-mask to endotracheal intubation and intermittent positive pressure ventilation with full ventilatory support.
8. External cardiac massage.

In all cases of acute cardiorespiratory compromise prompt and efficient treatment is mandatory and will prevent any harm to mother or baby, as soon as the mother has been resuscitated and is stable, the baby will usually be delivered by Caesarean section. The mother will continue to be ventilated until the effect of the local anaesthetic block has regressed.

Systemic toxic reaction

A systemic toxic reaction is caused by an excess level of local anaesthetic in the circulation. This occurs when the absorption of local anaesthetic into the tissues is greater than its rate of destruction.

The possible causes are as follows:

- excessive volume and/or concentration of local anaesthetic
- local anaesthetic administered too quickly or too frequently
- local anaesthetic absorbed rapidly into the circulation, for example by accidental intravenous injection or due to increased vascularity in the epidural space.

To avoid simple errors, all doses of local anaesthetic should be carefully checked and the safe maximum dose should not be exceeded except in exceptional circumstances (see Chapter 5). Accidental intravenous injection of local anaesthetic can only be avoided by careful technique. The severity of the reaction depends upon the blood level of local anaesthetic attained. Systemic toxic reactions are classified as mild, moderate or severe depending upon the blood level of local anaesthetic. The main points in diagnosing the severity of the reaction are as shown in Table 10.1. In the event of a massive overdose the local anaesthetic acts as a central nervous system depressant. This depresses the cardiorespiratory centres in the medulla, with consequent cardiorespiratory arrest.

Table 10.1 Severity of systemic toxic reaction

Mild	Moderate	Severe
circumoral tingling	confusion	hypoxia
tinnitus	slurred speech	hypotension
blurred vision	muscle twitching	loss of consciousness
nausea		convulsions
drowsiness		cardiac arrest

Treatment of systemic toxic reactions

Mild and moderate reactions

Careful observation and the administration of oxygen until the reaction subsides is usually all that is required.

Severe reactions

If convulsions occur, treatment is aimed at preventing maternal and fetal hypoxia. This is achieved by carrying out the following procedures.

1. **Oxygenate:**
   (a) maintain an airway
   (b) give oxygen initially via a face-mask and proceed if necessary to intermittent positive pressure ventilation via an endotracheal tube facilitated with sodium thiopentone and suxamethonium.
2. **Stop the fits:**
   give an anticonvulsant (lorazepam or thiopentone intravenously in sufficient doses to stop the convulsions).
3. **Maintain cardiac output:**
   (a) ensure that the wedge is in place to displace the gravid uterus from the major vessels at all times
   (b) give intravenous fluids
   (c) give external cardiac massage if necessary.

As a systemic toxic reaction can occur unexpectedly, full facilities for rapid resuscitation should always be readily available when performing or topping up an epidural.

Administering the wrong solution

Injecting the wrong solution through the epidural catheter into the epidural space is the error that should never occur, but unfortunately occasionally does with potentially disastrous results. The most effective way of preventing such an occurrence is to develop a routine of careful labelling and checking of the solution to be injected. A complaint by the patient of a sensation of pain or burning during injection should alert the anaesthetist that all is not well.

The solutions that have been injected in error are phenol, alcohol, contaminated solutions of local anaesthetic, potassium chloride and even ether. All can cause serious problems, which can be long lasting (see neurological deficit below).

Horner's syndrome

Horner's syndrome is a rare occurrence believed to be caused when some local anaesthetic in the epidural space reaches the level of the cervical sympathetic chain. The syndrome is unilateral and is diagnosed by the presence of the following signs on the affected side:

1. constriction of the pupil (myosis)
2. drooping of the eyelid (ptosis)
3. slight retraction of the globe of the eye into the orbit (enophthalmus)
4. loss of sweating on the side of the face (anhydrosis).

Horner's syndrome is an enigma in that it usually occurs as an isolated phenomenon during an otherwise normal epidural, although a not uncommon association is that the block achieved by the epidural may be observed to be unilateral. If it were simply caused by an ascending cervical block due to local anaesthetic solution tracking up the epidural space, it would be accompanied by a profound drop in blood pressure, but this does not happen.

The only clinical significance of the syndrome is in the anxiety caused to the patient because of her temporary altered facial appearance. All that is needed is reassurance that the effects will quickly wear off.

Postpartum problems with epidurals

The anaesthetist is frequently called to a variety of complaints in the puerperium and he or she must be able to diagnose with some confidence the problems that have been caused by an epidural and be able to give sound advice as to how to manage the patient.

The complaints vary considerably in their severity, significance and urgency, and therefore a rational method of dealing with them is necessary. This can only be achieved by first having a full understanding of the most common problems and their differential diagnoses.

Difficulty with removal of the epidural catheter

Normally the epidural catheter can be removed from the patient without difficulty. It should always be checked for completeness (see above).

Occasionally resistance may be felt when attempting to remove the catheter. A simple remedy is to place the woman in the same position she was in when the catheter was inserted and it is often found that the catheter will slide out easily. The epidural catheter must never be forcibly removed, if there is any difficultly the anaesthetist should attend.

Headache

This is discussed Chapter 11.

Backache

Backache after childbirth is common and has many possible causes. The precise relationship between epidurals and backache is not well defined, but the anaesthetist may be called to any patient with backache who has also had an epidural. The following facts may help to elucidate the cause.

The complaint of backache in all women in the childbearing age group is common – at any one time some 15–20% will currently complain of backache and 40% will admit to having suffered from it in the previous 9 months.

Fifty per cent of pregnant women will suffer backache at some stage during their pregnancy sufficient to alter their lifestyle. There are a large variety of causes including the following:

- fatigue
- increased joint mobility (due to lax ligaments caused by the increased levels of progesterone in pregnancy)
- hormonal effects – an increase in progestogen causes collagen fibres to have a greater volume, which can cause pressure on pain-sensitive structures (for example lateral cutaneous nerve of thigh)
- weight gain – increases the load to be carried by the spine
- posture (exaggerated lumbar lordosis)
- pressure on the spine from an enlarging uterus.

Epidurals and backache

A recent Cochrane review found no link between long-term backache and epidural insertion.

Causes directly attributable to epidurals are as follows:

- epidural haematoma
- epidural abscess
- bruising.

Perineal pain

Perineal pain is often thought to be greater after childbirth with an epidural. The epidural itself does not cause perineal pain but other coincidental factors may have this effect.

Forceps delivery

Forceps delivery usually requires an episiotomy, which can be painful in the puerperium. It is wrong to assume that the epidural is the reason for the forceps delivery. The indication for the epidural (for example malpresentation) may be the reason.

Sutures too tight

Episiotomies sutured under epidural analgesia do not need local anaesthetic infiltration and so the sutures may be tied more tightly as there is less perineal oedema.

Pain tolerance

It has been suggested anecdotally that women who have had a pain-free labour under epidural analgesia may be less tolerant of pain in the puerperium.

Neurological deficit

Any complaint of neurological deficit in the postpartum period should be responded to promptly in order to reach an accurate diagnosis, particularly to exclude urgent problems, give the correct treatment or advice, and reassure the patient. Neurological problems may be caused by childbirth itself or they may be due to the epidural.

The possible causes of neurological problems are as follows:

1. peripheral nerve lesions
2. epidural haematoma
3. epidural abcess
4. spinal artery occlusion
5. arachnoiditis
6. delayed recovery from the epidural.

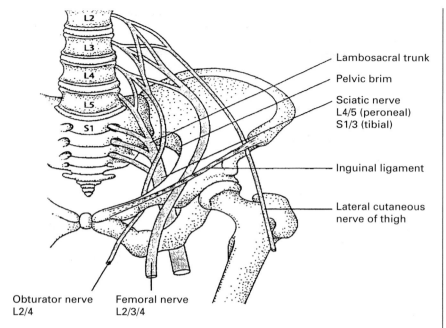

Lambosacral trunk

Pelvic brim

Sciatic nerve
L4/5 (peroneal)
S1/3 (tibial)

Inguinal ligament

Lateral cutaneous
nerve of thigh

Obturator nerve
L2/4

Femoral nerve
L2/3/4

Figure 10.1 Nerves and nerve trunks (from Holdcroft & Thomas, 1999, reproduced with permission from Blackwell Science)

Peripheral nerve lesions

Patients with peripheral nerve lesions complain of a variety of symptoms, such as areas of numbness on their legs or inability to move their legs properly. It is important to differentiate between symptoms of damage to a nerve root in the epidural space and symptoms of damage to a peripheral nerve. See Fig. 10.1.

Peripheral nerve damage due to obstetric causes

This normally involves more than one nerve root. The commonly damaged nerves in obstetrics are as follows.

1. **The lateral popliteal nerve (L2–3)** is usually damaged by the stirrups, which produce pressure at the head of the fibula. This causes foot drop.
2. **The lateral cutaneous nerve of the thigh (L2–3)** is usually damaged by swelling or pressure in the groin caused by the lithotomy position or simply the stretching caused by the gravid uterus. The effect is numbness on the antero-lateral aspect of the thigh.
3. **The femoral nerve (L2–3–4)** or **the sciatic nerve (L4–5/S1–3)** can be damaged by the lithotomy position. The effects are as follows:
   - femoral nerve – weak quadriceps, loss of knee reflex, hypoalgesia over the anterior aspect of the thigh

- sciatic nerve – sciatica (sciatic nerve damage can also be due to a disc protrusion).
4. **The sacral plexus nerve (L4–5/S1–4)** and **the obturator nerve (L5–S2)** both cross the pelvic brim and can be damaged by the passage of the fetal head or during forceps delivery. The effect is to upset bladder function, causing either retention of urine or loss of normal bladder sensation. It is important to note that bladder dysfunction can be due to obstetric causes rather than assuming that it is due to the epidural.

Peripheral nerve damage caused by the epidural

Symptoms are usually localized to the area supplied by one nerve root that has been pierced or abraded by the epidural catheter (for example an area of paraesthesia in one dermatome). The patient can be reassured that the symptoms will gradually disappear on their own as the damage heals. Very occasionally a more serious complication occurs when the epidural catheter becomes wrapped round a nerve root, which is then severed when the catheter is withdrawn.

Epidural haematoma

The occurrence of an epidural haematoma is a very rare but serious complication requiring immediate diagnosis and urgent intervention. The haematoma results from abnormal bleeding in the epidural space. If left unchecked, this collection of blood will compress nerve roots and eventually the spinal cord as the epidural space is enclosed.

The presence of an epidural haematoma should be suspected if the effects of an epidural have not worn off within 8 hours of the last 'top-up'. This suspicion will be heightened by finding a severe and usually symmetrical neurological deficit in the lower limbs and accompanied by sensory and motor loss and reflex changes. Diagnosis will be confirmed by urgent magnetic resonance imaging.

If the spinal cord is compressed, permanent neurological damage will result unless the haematoma is evacuated by laminectomy within 24–48 hours of its occurrence. Therefore whenever this condition is suspected, careful examination and early referral to a neurologist are vital.

Epidural abscess

An epidural abscess will produce the same symptoms as an epidural haematoma with the addition of the following symptoms:

- pain
- fever
- localized tenderness
- neck stiffness.

Investigation will show the following:

- increased white blood cell count
- protein and leucocytosis in the CSF.

Infection in the epidural space may be endogenous (for example from the transient bacteraemia associated with childbirth) or exogenous (from needles, solutions, etc.). Whatever the cause, it is a serious condition requiring urgent treatment with antibiotics. In some cases surgical evaluation of the abscess may be necessary.

Spinal artery occlusion

Occlusion of the spinal artery is a rare problem, which can occur when there is interference in the blood supply to the spinal cord. This may be caused by the following:

- reduction in arterial blood pressure
- venous engorgement.

Both these conditions can lead to a decreased blood flow in the spinal arteries, which in turn can cause ischaemia in the anterior two-thirds of the spinal cord. The effect of this is weakness in the lower part of the legs. Any sensory loss present is patchy and is due to associated ischaemia of the posterior roots. The problem is usually associated with an atherosclerotic vasculature, a condition not commonly seen in women of childbearing age.

The use of adrenaline in the epidural space increases the possibility of spinal artery occlusion by reducing arterial blood flow.

Arachnoiditis

Arachnoiditis is inflammation of the arachnoid membrane. It may or may not be associated with neurological damage. Possible causes of arachnoiditis are as follows:

- chemical contaminants in the epidural space (for example iodine, chlorhexidine, starch, potassium chloride)
- infection in the epidural space.

Chemical contamination is the most common cause of arachnoiditis, and for this reason any solutions introduced into the epidural space should be carefully checked, should be preservative free, and should be introduced through a bacterial filter.

Arachnoiditis can occur as an immediate consequence of bacterial infection in the epidural space. Tuberculous infection should be excluded where the onset of arachnoiditis is gradual.

The presenting symptom of arachnoiditis is back pain. This is caused by traction on the nervous tissue where it becomes adherent to the inflamed arachnoid membrane in the epidural space. Permanent neurological damage may result.

Treatment depends upon the cause. Unfortunately, there is no effective treatment for the condition where the cause is chemical contamination and so the emphasis is on prevention.

Delayed recovery from the epidural

Delayed recovery from the epidural anaesthetic is the most benign form of neurological complication. Normally the anaesthetic has worn off within eight hours, but it may take much longer in a few patients. It is usually a diagnosis of exclusion, other more serious causes having been considered first.

Headaches, dural puncture and epidural blood patching

Postpartum headache

This is a frequent complaint, and in the literature its incidence is reported as being between 8–25% in the early puerperium.

The woman who has also had an epidural is likely to have her headache attributed to that cause and the anaesthetist will be summoned. Whilst the headache may be due to a dural puncture, an occurrence the anaesthetist must be able to diagnose with confidence, a differential diagnosis of simple headache, cerebrovascular accident, cerebral tumour and meningitis may need to be considered. Therefore a careful history and examination of the woman is essential. Before discussing the diagnosis and management of dural puncture it should be stressed that good, carefully supervised teaching is essential to keep the incidence to a minimum. Wherever it takes place, the teaching of epidurals should be carefully supervised.

The diagnosis of dural puncture is usually made by the anaesthetist during insertion of the epidural, or may be obvious from the epidural record. It is very helpful if this is clear with full mention of any difficulties encountered during insertion. There are occasions when it only comes to light with the onset of a headache (and possibly other symptoms described below) in the puerperium.

Diagnosis of a post-dural puncture headache

The headache associated with dural puncture has the following characteristics.

- **Postural**. The headache is relieved by lying flat and is made worse by sitting up or standing. The leakage of CSF through the dural puncture causes a drop in the CSF pressure, which in turn produces traction on the dura, tentorium and blood vessels, all of which are sensitive to pain. The traction on these tissues, and therefore the headache, is greatest in the upright posture.

- **Occipital**. The headache is mainly occipital but can radiate to the frontal area.
- **Neck stiffness**. The woman often complains of a painful stiff neck, which is more comfortable in the supine position.
- **Vomiting**. A severe dural-puncture headache may be associated with vomiting.
- **Photophobia**. Photophobia is also associated with a severe dural-puncture headache.
- **Diplopia**. Diplopia is rarely complained of, but when present it is due to a sixth nerve palsy. This is thought to be due to traction on the meninges as a result of loss of CSF.

On examination, the woman with mild symptoms may be found to be ambulant and active, but with severe symptoms she will be at best just miserable and at worst severely incapacitated. The following signs should be looked for:

- meningism
- limited straight leg raising
- apyrexia (a negative finding, which may exclude meningitis).

In addition, it is recommended that a full neurological examination is carried out to exclude intracerebral pathology such as cerebrovascular accident, tumour or meningitis.

Dural puncture

This occurs when the epidural needle has travelled too far into the epidural space and punctured the dura leading to backflow or leakage of CSF. The incidence of is between 0.5–2% of epidurals depending upon the experience of the anaesthetist.

If the dural puncture occurs during insertion of the epidural needle there is usually no doubt about the diagnosis. However, if the epidural catheter threads through the dura into the CSF the diagnosis may not be so obvious, particularly if a closed-end catheter is used. If there is any doubt, the woman should be treated as though a dural puncture has occurred.

It is unlikely that the catheter alone is capable of puncturing the dura unless a defect has already been created by the epidural needle. Even when the anaesthetist is sure that no such defect has been caused, the tell-tale signs of CSF in the catheter should never be ignored as the consequences may be disastrous (see Chapter 10).

The event of dural puncture should always be recorded in the woman's records and a full explanation should be given to the woman and her partner. In order to minimize the effects of accidental dural puncture it is good policy to have a protocol of procedures to follow after the event. This will ensure good management and communication.

The aim of treatment is first to reduce the incidence of subsequent headache when the dural puncture is diagnosed at the time it happens, and second to alleviate symptoms when they develop either in those already diagnosed or in those diagnosed later in the puerperium.

Management of dural puncture

During labour

- Site the epidural at an adjacent space. Seek more senior help if appropriate.
- Inform the woman, the midwife and the obstetrician that a dural puncture has occurred.
- Clear documentation of the dural puncture is essential.
- Increase intravenous fluid to avoid dehydration.
- Avoid sudden movements if possible.
- Give epidural saline following delivery.

It is possible to leave an intrathecally placed catheter *in situ* and use it for the duration of labour and delivery. This requires meticulous care and communication between anaesthetist, midwife and obstetrician must be excellent. The intrathecal catheter can provide excellent analgesia and anaesthesia if required. All top-ups must be given by the anaesthetist.

Leaving the catheter *in situ* may reduce the incidence of post-dural puncture headache but this must be weighed against the ever present risk that a large volume of local anaesthetic will inadvertently be administered intrathecally leading to serious complications. (See Chapters 5 and 10)

Postpartum

Most women with a headache due to dural puncture have mild symptoms and require no treatment. However, it is most important that the woman is firmly reassured from the beginning that a dural puncture is neither a serious nor a life-threatening condition. If she has neck stiffness it should be stressed that this is not due to meningitis (after appropriate examination has first convinced the anaesthetist that this is the case). She should be told that the headache is usually short-lived – it rarely lasts more than six days, although in some women it may last for several weeks.

In all cases of dural puncture daily examination of the mother is strongly advised both to assess the onset of symptoms and to exclude the development of serious complications such as meningitis. If no advice or treatment is offered 70–80% of women will develop a headache to some degree.

Bed rest

It has been traditional practice to recommend 24 hours bed rest after dural puncture with the rationale that this reduces CSF pressure thus encouraging the puncture to heal more quickly. Research has shown that this has no value in reducing the incidence or duration of headache. It is still widely adopted for those women with headaches as a commonsense measure.

Analgesia

Choose simple analgesics that avoid constipation (for example paracetamol or diclofenac).

Fluids

The woman should be encouraged to drink plenty of fluids (to avoid dehydration).

Avoid straining

Lactulose may be prescribed to ensure gentle bowel action and the woman should be discouraged from bending or lifting until the headache resolves.

Caffeine

An intravenous infusion of caffeine sodium benzoate 0.5% has been described as beneficial in the treatment of dural-puncture headache. It is believed to work by preventing cerebral vasodilatation. It is not commonly used.

Epidural saline

A slow bolus of 50–100 ml normal saline administered into the epidural space prior to removal of the catheter reduces the incidence of post-dural puncture headache. This can be repeated six hourly if the catheter remains in place.

Alternatively an infusion of saline into the epidural space for 12–24 hours will reduce the incidence of headache by 12–30%. Preservative-free normal saline is used, delivered via a standard giving set connected to the bacterial filter attached to the epidural catheter. The giving set is run in the open position, allowing gravity to direct the rate of infusion. An infusion pump must not be used. The amount of saline infused in this way varies from about 50–500 ml per 12-hour period.

A complication of either approach is that the presence of normal saline in the epidural space may itself produce a sensation of pain in the back (most commonly between the shoulder blades), necessitating the cessation of the treatment.

Neither approach is as successful as epidural blood patching.

Epidural blood patching

Blood patching is a procedure where a sample of the woman's venous blood is injected into the epidural space at the site of the dural puncture to seal the leak of CSF. It is an invasive technique with undoubted effectiveness (over 70%), but carries with it further risks of complications.

Complications of blood patching

Blood in the epidural space is known to cause problems as is evidenced by the fact that during the operation of laminectomy meticulous care is taken to keep the nerve roots free from blood.

The potential complications of blood patching can be divided into immediate and long-term problems.

Immediate problems:

- failure
- dural puncture
- infection (blood is an ideal culture medium)
- arachnoiditis
- radiculitis
- cauda equina syndrome.

Long-term problems:

- fibrous bands
- obliteration of the epidural space
- problems with the next epidural.

Discussion of the merits of blood patching

Blood patching is effective in the treatment of dural puncture. Therefore the questions that arise are why this technique is not used routinely for all dural punctures and why there are reservations concerning its use even in women with severe symptoms

Immediate post-delivery routine use of blood patching

Points for:

Easy

There is already an epidural catheter in place through which to carry out the blood patch.

Mobility

She can participate in normal post natal activities without restriction (although she still may develop a headache).

Points against:

Unnecessary

Eighty-five per cent of dural-puncture headaches can be successfully treated by simple non-invasive measures. Routine blood patching would expose these women unnecessarily to the risks associated with blood patching.

Infection

At the time of childbirth there is normally a significant bacteraemia and this may increase the risk of infection being introduced to the epidural space via the blood patching sample.

Dilution

The blood-patching sample may be diluted in the epidural space by the local anaesthetic still present.

Site

Immediate blood patching would be carried out via the epidural catheter in place at the interspinous space adjacent to that used for the original epidural, which caused the dural puncture. Therefore the blood patch will not be at the site of the dural puncture.

Effectiveness

Blood patching performed immediately may not succeed in sealing the dural puncture, necessitating a repeat of the procedure.

Selective use of blood patching

The reason for selective use of blood patching is that it is an invasive procedure not without risks of complications, as has been discussed above. Therefore it may be thought not to be justifiable as a treatment for a headache which is not life-threatening, is self-limiting and usually resolves within six days. However, a woman with a severe dural-puncture headache may be confined to bed for several days, which may increase her risk of developing a deep vein thrombosis and subsequent pulmonary embolus. Less seriously, it is far from ideal for a mother to have a persistent headache in the first few days after childbirth, robbing her of the capacity to enjoy her baby at this important time.

How to perform a blood patch

1. Explain the procedure and the reason for doing it to the woman.
2. Obtain consent for the procedure.

3. Position the woman as for performing an epidural, women usually prefer the left-lateral position.
4. Find the epidural space at the level of the dural puncture and insert an epidural needle into the epidural space (see Chapter 3).
5. At the same time an assistant takes 20 ml of venous blood from the woman under sterile conditions. This sample is handed to the anaesthetist performing the blood patching.
6. A further 20 ml sample of venous blood is taken by the assistant for blood culture.
7. Inject the 20 ml sample of venous blood slowly into the epidural space via the epidural needle. If pain or paraesthesia is experienced by the woman during the injection, it should be temporarily stopped and then cautiously continued. Dizziness and tinnitus are occasionally experienced by the woman during this injection.
8. Remove the epidural needle as soon as the epidural injection of blood has been completed and apply a dressing.
9. Instruct the woman to lie flat for about 30–60 minutes, preferably with her knees raised to flatten the lumbar lordosis.
10. The woman should be able to get up and resume her normal activities after about 60 minutes and she should find that her headache has been completely relieved.

Follow-up

All women who have had or who are suspected of having had an accidental dural puncture should be followed by the anaesthetic team after discharge from hospital. Ideally a clinic appointment for around six weeks after delivery should be arranged to ensure that any problems have resolved. The woman can be debriefed appropriately and given advice for the next pregnancy.

Summary of management of dural-puncture headache

- Prevention of accidental dural puncture by teaching of junior doctors should be a priority.
- Simple non-invasive treatments are successful in 85% of cases.
- The benefits of invasive treatments should be carefully weighed against side-effects and complications.
- Any headache where there is doubt about the aetiology needs careful consultation with a neurologist.
- Careful follow-up is required in all cases of suspected accidental dural puncture.

12 Regional anaesthesia for lower-segment Caesarean section

General anaesthesia continues to carry a significant risk of maternal mortality, in part because the physiological and anatomical changes associated with pregnancy render the pregnant woman more prone to difficulties with intubation, hypoxia and aspiration. Therefore the move towards regional anaesthetic techniques and the development of obstetric anaesthetic services in recent years has played a significant part in reducing maternal mortality. This is well documented in the CEMACH reports.

Regional anaesthesia is now established as the routine anaesthetic for Caesarean section, and when carefully performed it provides safe anaesthesia for both mother and baby allowing both the mother and her partner to be involved in the birth. Regional anaesthesia for lower-segment Caesarean section is provided by the epidural or spinal routes or a combination of these as the combined spinal epidural (CSE). The particular technique employed depends on the clinical scenario, the anaesthetist's preference and the mother's choice. It must be emphasized that a working epidural in labour can rapidly enable anaesthesia for an emergency Caesarean section, thus reducing the need for hastily sited blocks or general anaesthesia.

In this chapter regional anaesthesia for elective and for emergency Caesarean section is described. There are some situations in which regional anaesthesia is not appropriate, such as maternal refusal, a contraindication to regional anaesthesia and massive haemorrhage. Detailed discussion is outside the scope of this book.

Urgency of Caesarean section is classified as shown in Table 12.1.

This classification is helpful for audit and ensuring that the really urgent Caesarean sections are performed in good time. There are very few occasions where the baby needs to be delivered as fast as possible. The delivery-suite team must communicate well to ensure that women are given the safest anaesthetic option for mother and baby.

The choice of anaesthesia for a Caesarean section is dependent on a clear communication of the urgency of the Caesarean section. The anaesthetist should have a clear understanding of the clinical condition of both mother and baby. Regular ward rounds should ensure that the anaesthetist is aware of potential problems. Ideally the communication should be clear and concise and occur between the obstetrician and the anaesthetist.

Table 12.1 Urgency of Caesarean section

Grade 1	Emergency	Immediate threat to life of woman or fetus
Grade 2	Urgent	Maternal or fetal compromise, which is not immediately life threatening
Grade 3	Scheduled	Needing early delivery but no maternal or fetal compromise
Grade 4	Elective	At a time to suit the woman and the maternity team

Regional anaesthetic techniques

A regional block that provides surgical anaesthesia for a lower-segment Caesarean section requires a more extensive and a more profound block than one for analgesia in labour. The block must be sufficient to anaesthetize each of the layers between skin and uterus. These layers comprise the following:

- skin
- subcutaneous tissue
- rectus sheath
- rectus abdominus muscle
- abdominal peritoneum
- visceral peritoneum
- uterus.

The most sensitive of these layers is the abdominal peritoneum, which requires a block extending at least up to the level of T4. The full extent of the block should be from T4–S4. The extent of the block should be tested both to cold, usually using ethyl chloride spray, and to touch, using a sharp needle such as the Neuropen. A block to light touch up to T5 has also been suggested. Each dermatome should be tested to ensure that the block is not patchy and particular attention should be paid to the height of the block to touch. Inadequate anaesthesia will result in the mother feeling pain and this may well lead to post-traumatic stress and litigation.

The practical techniques for siting regional blockade are described in Chapters 3 and 4.

Spinal and CSE anaesthesia

Spinal and CSE anaesthesia are common techniques of regional anaesthesia for Caesarean section. These are further described in Chapter 4. Spinal anaesthesia is a 'one-shot' technique for producing regional anaesthesia, which has a rapid onset of action and a limited duration. These properties are ideal when the need arises for an anaesthetic for an emergency Caesarean section. Spinal and CSE anaesthesia are both used for grade 2, 3 and 4 Caesarean sections where there is no working epidural *in situ.* The choice of anaesthesia for a grade 1 Caesarean section will depend on the clinical condition of the patient and baby and the experience of the operator. There are many grade 1 Caesarean sections where a spinal may be the anaesthetic of choice.

Other indications are as a means for avoiding a general anaesthetic for a short obstetric procedure, perhaps where there is not already an epidural running. (See Chapter 8.)

Epidural anaesthesia

An epidural that is providing good analgesia in labour can be topped up and be ready for an emergency (grade 1, 2 or 3) Caesarean section in a relatively short time. This is most easily done if:

- the epidural has been kept well topped up throughout labour
- there is good communication between and team involvement of the obstetrician, the midwife and the anaesthetist
- forewarned about the possibility of Caesarean section, the anaesthetist can take particular care with the top-ups throughout labour.

Epidural anaesthesia has a very limited place for elective (grade 4) Caesarean sections as the onset of the block can be slow and there is sometimes difficulty in achieving a profound surgical block, particularly in the sacral segments. Epidural anaesthesia was the regional anaesthetic of choice before the advent of CSE for patients in whom cardiovascular stability was essential.

Topping up an epidural for Caesarean section

Once the decision has been made to proceed to an emergency Caesarean section the anaesthetist must rapidly go through a checklist designed to produce surgical anaesthesia as soon as possible.

1. Find out how urgent the impending Caesarean section is.
2. Check the height of the block.
3. Extend the block from T4 to the sacral roots:
   - check the level of the block
   - check when the last top-up was given
   - calculate and give the top-up for Caesarean section.

If delivery is very urgent, the woman may be transferred to the operating theatre immediately after the top-up for Caesarean section has been given provided that the anaesthetist supervises the move closely. Intravenous fluids and lateral tilt should all be employed during the transfer and oxygen, ephedrine and CTG monitoring should be readily available.

Once the patient is on the operating table, a final assessment of the adequacy of the block will determine whether an emergency general anaesthetic should be administered or whether the obstetrician can proceed with the Caesarean section under epidural anaesthesia.

Talking the woman through these events is rarely a problem as she is usually relieved that a difficult labour is about to come to an end, and as a rule she is motivated to remain awake and see and enjoy the childbirth with her partner.

Extending the block

For completeness two safe recipes are described below. Both the mixtures described are usually mixed with opiate, either fentanyl 50 µg or diamorphine 250 or 300 mg. These drugs are further described in Chapter 5.

Using bupivacaine 0.5%

A dose of 15–20 ml of bupivacaine 0.5% will usually produce a block suitable for Caesarean section after at least 20 minutes. If more is required, the toxic dose (2–3.5 mg/kg) should only be exceeded in exceptional circumstances. The motor block produced by bupivacaine 0.5% is profound.

Method

1. 10 ml bupivacaine 0.5% is given with the patient in the left-lateral position.
2. After 5 minutes the patient is turned and a further 5 ml bupivacaine 0.5% is given in the right-lateral position.
3. Blood pressure is checked at 5, 10, 15 and 20 minutes, and at any time that the patient's condition causes concern. Ephedrine and intravenous fluid should be readily available to treat hypotension.
4. The block is assessed 20 minutes after the initial dose:
   - block at or above T4 and extending to the sacral roots – EPIDURAL IS READY.
   - block below T4 – extend the block upwards by giving additional dose of bupivacaine 0.5%, the amount depending upon the level of the block and the weight of the patient. Keep the patient horizontal, left- or right-lateral. Consider some head-down tilt. Consider conversion to general anaesthesia.
   - block at or above T4 but inadequate for the sacral roots – sit the patient up and give a further dose of bupivacaine 0.5%.

Using lidocaine 2% with 1:200 000 adrenaline

The local anaesthetic solution is made up with 20 ml of lidocaine 2% plus 0.1 ml of 1:1000 adrenaline, which produces the required dilution of 1:200 000 adrenaline. The adrenaline should be freshly mixed with the lidocaine. The method of administration is similar to that for bupivacaine. If more than a total of 20 ml of local anaesthetic is required, lidocaine 2% without adrenaline should be used. The toxic dose (7 mg/kg) should not be exceeded.

Peri-operative management

Pre-operative management

It is vitally important that the mother is given information about the anaesthetic for the Caesarean section at the earliest opportunity. As over one-fifth of mothers have a Caesarean section, the best time for this is in the antenatal period. For further information see Chapter 1.

The anaesthetist should visit the woman and perform the routine history and examination as for any anaesthetic. In addition to this an obstetric and past obstetric history should be ascertained. Consent must be taken for the anaesthetic procedure(s) undertaken.

It is important that all women that are at risk or planned to have a Caesarean section are given appropriate antacid therapy, such as ranitidine.

Investigations
Full blood count (FBC) as minimum, others as indicated.

Intra-operative management

A Caesarean section is a major abdominal operation, and often comes as an emergency when the mother has already been drained by hours of labour.

Whatever the circumstances of the Caesarean section, a quiet and supportive environment should be maintained to enable the mother to have the best experience possible.

The standards of care must be the same as for any other operating theatre, full monitoring should be applied before regional blockade and used at all times. The anaesthetist should remain with the woman at all times to ensure her safety.

The woman should be accompanied by the midwife at all times, CTG monitoring should be used, particularly once a regional block for anaesthesia has been instituted, as this is a time of potentially profound cardiovascular compromise for the mother.

Positioning the patient on the operating table

Careful positioning of the patient on the operating table will prevent avoidable problems during surgery. The main points are lateral tilt, the position of the head and shoulders, and elevation of the head-end of the table.

Lateral tilt

The weight of the gravid uterus must be displaced from the aorta and inferior vena cava at all times to avoid aorto-caval compression. The most practical way to achieve this is to tilt the operating table electronically though if this is not possible then a 15° wedge can be used or the patient's buttock can be elevated with a litre bag of intravenous fluid. The anaesthetist should personally check that the wedge is in a good position (Fig. 12.1).

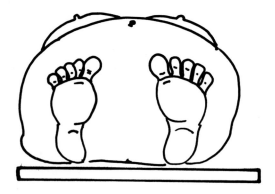

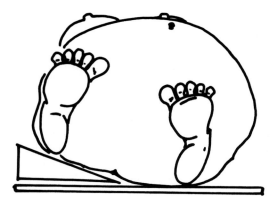

Figure 12.1 Demonstration of the wedged position (a) unwedged, (b) wedged

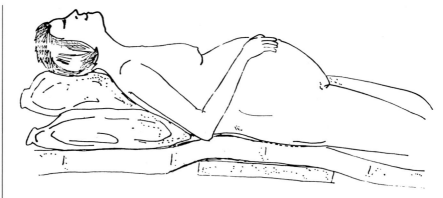

Figure 12.2 Position on the operating table for Caesarean section

Position of the head and shoulders
The patient's head and shoulders should be comfortably supported on pillows to allow free and easy breathing. The position should also be suitable for intubation should that be necessary in an emergency.

Elevation of the head-end of the table
A gentle slope from head to pelvis helps to prevent blood and body fluids from tracking up the paracolic gutters. These fluids could cause peritoneal irritation under the diaphragm, which may not be adequately anaesthetized by the regional block. The slope should not be so steep as to cause pooling of blood in the legs, nor should there be undue strain on the patient's spine.

Making sure that the patient is well positioned and comfortable can be tedious, but it is most important for her well-being throughout the operation. Once positioned (Fig. 12.2) she cannot be moved until after the Caesarean section has been performed.

Organization of the drapes
Drapes are placed in such a way as to provide a screen between the patient's head and the operating site without detaching her from the proceedings.

Inviting the partner into the operating theatre
When the patient is stable and the drapes have been positioned, the partner may be invited and escorted into the operating theatre. The partner is best seated at the head-end of the table and it is prudent to have an understanding that they may leave if they wish or are requested to do so.

Delivery of the baby
The drapes should be lowered so that the couple can see their baby as it is delivered and ideally as recommended by the National Institute for Health

and Clinical Excellence (NICE) guidelines the baby should have skin-to-skin contact with the mother as soon as is safely possible.

Problems encountered

Problems during Caesarean section can be minimized by careful attention to detail and close observation and monitoring during the operation. When problems do occur rapid diagnosis and treatment is required. The anaesthetist should be prepared to accept failure and be ready to opt out and give a general anaesthetic at any stage. There is no place for 'patching up' a poor regional block with polypharmacy.

Hypotension

The most common cause for hypotension is inadequate lateral tilt, and when this is the case the blood pressure is rapidly restored when this is corrected. Supine hypotension should always be regarded as a potentially serious problem; if left untreated it could result in cardiac arrest. Its detection requires close observation of the patient with a quick response if she looks pale or feels nauseated or dizzy. Other possible causes of hypotension are extensive sympathetic block or severe blood loss. Severe blood loss (for example resulting from a torn uterine artery) demands urgent general anaesthesia before the patient collapses.

Treatment of hypotension should follow these logical steps.

- Check the position of the patient. Is she adequately wedged?
- Give intravenous fluid.
- Give oxygen by face-mask.
- Increase the rate of the phenylephrine infusion.
- Check the height of the block.

Nausea and vomiting

When nausea or vomiting occurs before surgery it is usually associated with hypotension. Therefore treatment is correction of the reason for hypotension as described above. During surgery it may be due to either hypotension, handling of the peritoneum or exteriorization of the uterus by the surgeon. Treatment is as follows.

- Check the blood pressure.
- Check for and correct supine hypotension.
- If blood pressure is low and not due to caval compression give intravenous fluids and increase the rate of the phenylephrine infusion or give ephedrine in 3 mg boluses.
- If nausea or vomiting is due to surgery inform the surgeon. Surgery under regional anaesthesia should always be gentle and the uterus should not be exteriorized, in line with NICE guidance.

- Consider giving intravenous anti-emetic for persistent nausea and vomiting.

Bradycardia

Bradycardia is usually associated with hypotension, particularly hypotension resulting from a block that extends too high (beyond T4; see Chapter 6). The treatment is almost the same as for hypotension.

- Check the position of the patient.
- Give intravenous fluid.
- If there is no improvement, give 3 mg ephedrine intravenously (repeat if necessary).
- If there is still no response, consider giving atropine 0.6 mg intravenously.
- Check the height of the block.

Difficulty in breathing

This is usually due to either apprehension or panic on the part of the patient or to a block that extends too high. Depending upon the nature of the problem, treatment is as follows.

- Reassure the patient.
- Give oxygen by face-mask.
- Check the adequacy of respiration (ability to cough, oxygen saturation).
- Check blood pressure and pulse.
- If respiration is significantly impaired, give emergency general anaesthetic.

The patient panics or feels pain

Feelings of panic by the patient are usually engendered by pain or discomfort due to an inadequate block. Even though the block has been tested just prior to surgery and is thought to be adequate, a complaint of pain cannot be ignored and should be particularly checked when the peritoneum is incised. Further analgesia or **conversion to a general anaesthetic** may need to be offered. It is important to document on the anaesthetic chart any complaint of pain, what solution was offered, and what was refused or accepted by the patient so that any future claim for compensation for an inadequate block can be countered. The flowchart shown in Fig. 12.3 gives a plan for dealing with panic.

Entonox

Entonox (50:50 nitrous oxide–oxygen mixture) may be sufficient to tide the patient over incision of the peritoneum or until other additional analgesia is being organized.

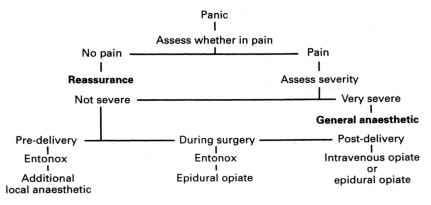

Figure 12.3 Flowchart showing procedure for dealing with panic

Epidural opiate
If there is an epidural *in situ* then further opiate may be given, either fentanyl or diamorphine.

Intravenous opiate
A small dose of intravenous opiate given just post-delivery of the baby produces excellent analgesia and a mild degree of euphoria and sedation without risk of significant respiratory depression or cardiovascular instability.

Additional epidural local anaesthetic
If an epidural is *in situ* then an incremental top-up may be given.

Post-operative management (recovery)

Observation

The woman needs to be cared for in an appropriate environment whilst she recovers from the effects of anaesthesia and surgery. The midwife or nurse should remain **with the woman** throughout this time. The woman should be fully monitored for at least 30 minutes according to Association of Anaesthetists of Great Britain and Ireland (AAGBI)/OAA guidelines. Routine post-Caesarean section observations should include the following:

- pulse
- blood pressure
- O_2 saturation
- respiratory rate
- sedation score
- temperature
- pain score

- wound check
- PV loss
- IV site
- drain
- urinary output
- patient colour
- leg power.

An example recovery observation chart is included in Appendix I.

Analgesia

A plan for post-operative analgesia should be in place, and the woman should be offered analgesia on a regular basis. Such as:

- paracetamol 1G QDS
- diclofenac 50 mg TDS PO or 100 mg BD PR for 72 hours (if no contraindication).

If the woman is in significant pain, consider

- giving epidural analgesia
- stronger oral analgesia
- patient-controlled analgesia (PCA) or IM morphine.

If intrathecal diamorphine has been used then regular observation should continue for a minimum of 8 hours. Systemic opiates should be avoided for 12–24 hours.

Nausea and vomiting should be treated promptly, intravenous cyclizine is usually effective.

Bonding

Skin-to-skin contact and commencement of breast feeding should be encouraged as soon as practically possible, in line with current NICE guidance.

13 Setting up and running an obstetric anaesthetic service

The need for an epidural service

The provision of pain relief in labour has historically been thwarted by superstition, religious bias and general mistrust, and it has probably only gained respectability in Western cultures following Queen Victoria's celebrated use of chloroform during childbirth in 1853. In the last 50 years Europe has experienced a significant fall in maternal mortality and morbidity, which, together with the development of effective pain relief techniques in labour, now gives every pregnant woman a high expectation of well-being for herself and her baby. Perhaps taking this expectation for granted, there is currently a swing towards natural childbirth with the minimum of intervention. Epidural analgesia may thus be perceived to be unnecessarily invasive and may not be offered.

The obstetric anaesthetist is often seen as an inserter of epidurals rather than the person best able to help a labouring woman cope with her pain openly and with dignity. It is the authors' view that the development of a pain-relief service in the delivery suite, run by an obstetric anaesthetist, is the best way to ensure that all women have a choice and can come to an informed decision about pain relief for their labour.

Obstetric anaesthetic practice began as an emergency anaesthetic service where general anaesthesia was often administered in far from ideal circumstances. This is clearly illustrated by successive Confidential Enquiries into Maternal Deaths, where anaesthesia has been shown to contribute significantly to maternal mortality. With the development of obstetric anaesthesia as a subspecialty and the introduction of epidural services, the mortality due to anaesthesia has fallen. The first report covered the triennium 1952–1954 and there were 49 deaths that were attributed to anaesthesia and 20 more where anaesthesia was contributory. Though the number of direct deaths due to anaesthesia has fallen dramatically there is no place for complacency, as 7 deaths solely attributable to anaesthesia were reported in the 2000–2002 report and there were a further 20 deaths where anaesthesia played a contributory role. General anaesthesia in pregnancy still kills fit healthy women, and its reduction is to be encouraged by the extensive use of epidural analgesia, and spinal and epidural anaesthesia. The safety of obstetric anaesthesia has already improved with the growth of epidural services, and this should continue as pain-relief services become established.

The epidural service

In the process of building up a comprehensive obstetric anaesthetic service the place of the availability of epidural analgesia can be evaluated by looking at the advantages and potential problems.

Advantages of the availability of epidural analgesia

1. Epidurals offer the best analgesia available.
2. They may be used for operative deliveries, thus reducing the need for general anaesthesia.
3. Stress-free labour is achieved owing to abolition of the pathological response to pain (pain causes reflex increase in the pulse rate, blood pressure, circulating catecholamines, ventilation rate, maternal acidosis and general level of anxiety). This may be particularly helpful where there are complex obstetric or medical problems (see Chapters 8 and 9).
4. There are benefits to the baby in a well-managed epidural as a result of the following effects.
   - Avoidance of hyperventilation in the mother. It has been shown that oxygenation is higher in babies born to mothers receiving epidural analgesia than in those where the mother has endured a painful labour.
   - Placental (intervillous) blood flow is usually improved (provided that the mother is well hydrated and supine hypotension is avoided by maintaining the lateral position).
   - Utero-placental blood flow is improved. The maternal stress response to a painful labour causes an increase in circulating catecholamines which reduces utero-placental perfusion. Epidural analgesia blocks this response.
   - Neurobehavioural scoring of the newborn is improved (compared with the neonate born to a distressed mother or to one who has had conventional analgesia).

Potential problems of epidural analgesia
Safety
The success of an epidural service depends on the maintenance of high standards of care to minimize complications from epidurals (see Chapters 10 and 11).

Cost
A 24-hour epidural service demands high staffing levels (doctors and midwives) to be effective. When the decision is made to set up an epidural service the management considerations are as follows:

- How much money is required?
- What staffing levels are needed (consultant anaesthetists, junior anaesthetists, midwives and support staff)?
- What is the expected workload?
- Is there sufficient work to justify setting up a service?

Recent reports have suggested that an obstetric unit should have at least 3000 deliveries per year for an epidural service to be viable. In smaller units cross-cover by the duty anaesthetist may jeopardize a 24-hour service (obstetric work is renowned for its unpredictability and for being scattered throughout 24 hours).

Thus the *need* for epidural services in obstetric units is well established, but there is also a broader need for more involvement of anaesthetists in the delivery suite. This can be identified in the following areas:

- pain relief
- anaesthesia
- management of the sick patient
- high dependency care on the labour ward.

Pain-relief service

To be effective a pain-relief service must include active involvement in all forms of pain relief:

- relaxation
- transcutaneous nerve stimulation (TENS)
- nitrous oxide (Entonox)
- pethidine by intramuscular route
- pethidine and other opioids by patient-controlled analgesia systems (PCAS)
- epidurals.

The role of the obstetric anaesthetist in a pain-relief service goes far beyond just 'putting in an epidural' and should include participation in education of the general public, parentcraft talks and teaching of nurses, midwives, technicians and medical staff, together with working as an active member of the delivery-room team. The aim is both to improve the safety of parturients and to provide comprehensive advice on analgesia and anaesthesia.

Anaesthesia

The provision of cover for an emergency anaesthetic service on an obstetric unit is the minimum basic requirement of an anaesthetic department. It is tempting for budget-conscious administrators and departmental heads to see this as their only requirement and to limit resources accordingly. This is short-sighted and is to be resisted. The development of a full 24-hour epidural service will dramatically reduce the need for urgent general anaesthesia in a delivery suite, thus bringing about significant improvements in maternal and neonatal morbidity and mortality.

Management of the sick patient

There are many occasions in a busy obstetric unit when seriously ill or collapsed patients have to be resuscitated and treated:

- pre-eclampsia/eclampsia
- severe haemorrhage
- pulmonary embolus
- amniotic fluid embolus
- cardiac arrest
- systemic infection or sepsis.

The obstetric anaesthetist is well placed to take an active part in immediate resuscitation for such problems and for the development of treatment protocols and staff training.

High-dependency care on the labour ward

The concept of a high-dependency unit or an intensive-therapy unit as part of an obstetric unit is a fairly recent development, and clearly the obstetric anaesthetist has a role in the management of the severely ill obstetric patient:

1. to improve the standard of post-operative care and pain relief (for example with the use of patient-controlled analgesia and epidural opiates)
2. to monitor carefully patients with medical problems (for example cardiac problems, diabetes)
3. to treat the severely ill obstetric patient (for example haemorrhage, pre-eclampsia/eclampsia).

The careful nursing and monitoring of these categories of patients together with an intensive medical input should improve the morbidity associated with them.

Setting up and running an epidural service

Once the need for a 24-hour epidural service has been firmly established, setting it up needs to be costed. This can best be done by identifying the resources that are considered essential under the following headings:

- staff
- accommodation
- equipment
- teaching
- record-keeping and audit.

Staff

Staffing an epidural service will not be achieved simply by the provision of a few extra trainee anaesthetists to cover the 24 hours. It can only be sustained by the support of a team that will include the following:

- consultant anaesthetic staff
- trainee anaesthetic staff
- midwifery staff
- trained assistance for the anaesthetist, for example operating department practitioners (ODP)
- secretarial staff.

High standards should be aimed for from the beginning, bearing in mind that the service will be required to operate 24 hours per day, 7 days per week, 365 days per year. There may well be occasions when staffing levels will be compromised, and when decisions have to be made to cut staff. It is well to remember that the service will only be as strong as its weakest link.

Consultant anaesthetic staff

Guidelines for the number of notional half-days that an obstetric unit will support is set out in the publication *OAA/AAGBI Guidelines for Anaesthetic Services* (revised edition 2005). The basic minimum recommended for a consultant-led obstetric unit is ten consultant anaesthetic sessions per week to allow for full 'working hours' consultant cover.

Ideally, more than one consultant anaesthetist should be involved in the obstetric unit in order to balance the workload (although too many can cause problems with cohesion within the unit!). The advantage of several anaesthetists sharing an interest in this work is that a specialist on-call rota can be organized without too onerous a workload for any one consultant.

Trainee and permanent non-consultant career grade anaesthetic staff

Trainee and non-consultant career grade anaesthetic staff are a vital element in maintaining a 24-hour epidural service, and so it is worthwhile having criteria for their attachment to the maternity unit. The important points are as follows:

- grade and/or experience
- job description, on-call duties.

Grade and/or experience

As a general principle the anaesthetist should have at least one year's experience in anaesthesia and success in the Primary FRCA examination. Although each anaesthetic department will set its own standards, approximately this level of experience is necessary to cope competently with the on-call commitment of the maternity unit. Individual assessment of each anaesthetist should also be taken into account.

Job description

The best arrangement is that the duties of trainee anaesthetic staff should be wholly confined to the maternity unit during their period of attachment or rotation. However, depending upon staffing levels and the size of the hospital, cover for the maternity unit may have to be shared with other commitments, for example intensive care or general on-call duties. Priorities may have to be worked out, but as a general principle a junior anaesthetist should not be left covering more than one unit at a time. A new junior obstetric anaesthetist should not be left alone on call before having received orientation to the unit and adequate teaching.

Midwifery staff

To run a safe epidural service the basic level of midwifery staffing should allow for a midwife to be in attendance with every woman who has an epidural in place. The ideal is that a midwife should constantly be with all labouring women. Insistence on this condition means that the number of epidurals performed may at times be limited by the number of midwives available.

An epidural service will be helped enormously if the midwives are enthusiastic and well informed about epidurals. The importance of midwifery teaching is discussed later in this chapter.

Trained assistant for the anaesthetist

The complement of trained operating department practitioners (ODPs) in the maternity unit should be sufficient to allow 24-hour cover. Their presence is particularly important for emergency work. Skilled assistance for the anaesthetist may be provided from the nursing grades, but an ODP is usually the best-trained person for the job. The permanent attachment of an ODP to a maternity unit brings other benefits, for example the maintenance of equipment and the teaching of midwifery staff.

Secretarial support

Planning and setting up an epidural service generates an administrative workload, which requires secretarial support. This may be provided by the main anaesthetic department, but in larger units an anaesthetic secretary designated to the maternity unit is an asset.

Accommodation

Minimum requirements are an office for the anaesthetic staff and a rest room for the duty anaesthetist equipped for rest and study. The office, which should be situated on the delivery suite, creates a home base for the anaesthetist from where administration, teaching, audit and research can be directed. The rest accommodation should be in close proximity to the delivery suite.

Equipment

The aim is that all equipment should be safe and reliable, and it is worth time and effort in selection and costing to achieve this. There are two categories of equipment:

• major items (capital expenditure)
• disposables and drugs (running costs).

Major items of equipment

The basic items required to carry out an epidural and to provide immediate resuscitation are as follows:

1. a tipping bed (allows head-down position)
2. suction apparatus
3. oxygen (cylinder or pipeline and means of administration)
4. wedge (or other means to allow 15° lateral tilt)
5. blood pressure monitor
6. anaesthetic machine (equipped for resuscitation and ventilation)
7. electrocardiograph monitor
8. cardiac arrest equipment (defibrillator and drugs).

Items 1–5 should be to hand in the patient's room, and items 6–8 should be readily available in the maternity unit. An 'epidural trolley' is a useful addition for convenient storage of disposable items and drugs in use.

Disposable items and drugs

All the items required for an epidural are fully listed and described in Chapter 3.

The disposable items can be supplied in two ways:

• individually supplied items backed up with a basic pack of towels, drapes and gowns from the hospital's central sterile supplies department.
• a 'tailor-made' pack containing all items necessary for an epidural supplied by a commercial firm.

In general, commercially available packs are more convenient and cost-effective for a small unit, and individually supplied items can work out cheaper for a large unit. The advantages of the latter are that more flexibility is possible, for example to change needle type, catheter type, etc., and dependence on one supplier is avoided. The final choice of equipment will depend upon individual requirements and preferences (see Chapter 3), the size of the unit and the cost of each item.

Drugs

An array of drugs is required for the following purposes.

1. Drugs for resuscitation and general anaesthesia. The drug cupboards in the anaesthetic room, the operating theatre and the delivery suite should all be well stocked. A full list of these drugs is beyond the scope of this book.
2. Drugs for injection into the epidural space.
   - Local anaesthetic agents: lignocaine 2%, bupivacaine 0.1% with fentanyl 2 μg/ml, bupivacaine or levobupivacaine 0.25% and 0.5%
   - Others: saline, opioids, ephedrine, atropine, phenyephrine, adrenaline, diamorphine.

All should be free from preservatives and additives.

Teaching

The most difficult aspect of running an epidural service is to achieve and maintain a high standard of care. The service will not succeed unless all the members of the delivery-suite team have a good understanding of epidurals. This can only be attained through a comprehensive teaching programme involving the following:

- medical staff: obstetricians, anaesthetists of all grades
- ODPs (assistants for the anaesthetists)
- midwives and student midwives
- parturients – as part of being given a balanced view of pain relief in labour.

Medical staff
Obstetricians

The support and close involvement of all grades of obstetricians (and paediatricians) is a prerequisite to running an effective epidural service. Formal and informal communication between anaesthetists and obstetricians is important as changes of practice in one discipline can affect the other. This cooperation should be particularly helpful to trainee grades as it will result in the use of guidelines for the delivery suite, which will include the place of epidurals.

Anaesthetists
A significant proportion of a consultant obstetric anaesthetist's work is a commitment to teaching the training grades of anaesthetists. The subject matter will cover all aspects of obstetric analgesia and anaesthesia including epidurals, with equal emphasis on the academic and the practical.

Practical instruction
The trainee new to obstetric anaesthesia should first be shown round the maternity unit and introduced to the staff. The initial practical instruction on the technique of inserting an epidural is best given in a general operating theatre, perhaps demonstrated on a surgical or gynaecological patient where an epidural forms an integral part of their anaesthetic management. This approach is less stressful to the teacher and the trainee than learning on an awake, anxious maternity patient. Towards the end of his or her attachment to the maternity unit the trainee will become more involved in the unit, and some may be sufficiently confident and competent to take part in on-call duties, although this is usually covered by an anaesthetist of specialist registrar grade.

The experienced trainee new to the maternity unit should be allowed a period of orientation and introduction to the unit's policy on the management of epidurals and their problems, and must be assessed as competent before being given the responsibility of on-call work. There should be good support from senior staff.

Academic teaching
This may take the form of lectures and tutorials as part of an FRCA course as well as opportunistic teaching during the period of attachment to the maternity unit. Wide reading on the subject – both textbooks and journals – is to be encouraged.

ODP/trained assistant for the anaesthetist
A programme of teaching and training for the ODP attached to the maternity unit will help him or her to play a vital role in maintaining high standards on the delivery suite, especially if they are a permanent member of staff. The ODP will be involved primarily in assisting the anaesthetist but will also maintain and order equipment and teach his or her own trainee staff, ensuring continuity of the service 24 hours a day.

Midwives
The role of the midwife is central to the smooth running and safety of an epidural service. For this reason epidural analgesia should be taught to

student midwives as an integral part of their lectures on pain relief and anaesthesia in obstetrics. The theoretical aspects should then be built on with practical instruction on the delivery suite whilst they are looking after labouring women who have an epidural in place. Midwives should also feel confident to discuss the subject knowledgeably with mothers.

The subject matter of a teaching programme for epidurals for midwives can be summarized as follows.

1. Indications and contraindications for epidurals (so that the midwife will be able to discuss and give advice on their use).
2. Anatomy of the epidural space.
3. How to assist the anaesthetist in performing an epidural. Discussion of the problems encountered by the anaesthetist.
4. Topping up epidurals.
5. Choice of local anaesthetic agent, including standard dosages and side-effects.
6. The effect of the epidural – what areas are blocked.
7. Physiological changes caused by the epidural and how this affects the mother and the fetus.
8. Management of labour with epidural analgesia.
9. Problems associated with epidural analgesia.
10. Resuscitation: all midwives, particularly those involved in an epidural service, should be competent in basic cardiopulmonary resuscitation in pregnancy and they should be able to assist the anaesthetist in advanced resuscitation. They should always know the whereabouts of cardiac arrest equipment.

In units where midwives are expected to top up epidurals additional instruction is required. The Nursing and Midwifery Council state their rules governing this practice in their *Handbook of Midwives Rules and Standards 2004*.

In simple terms, this means that specific teaching of midwives on topping up epidurals is required. Most hospitals in the United Kingdom issue a 'Certificate of competence for topping up epidurals' to midwives on completion of a course of instruction and a designated number of top-ups supervised by a consultant obstetric anaesthetist and a senior midwife.

Parturients

The importance of offering information on pain relief and epidurals to maternity patients throughout pregnancy is discussed in Chapter 1. The main aim of covering this topic in parentcraft classes is to give mothers-to-be the best possible chance of having a balanced view of pain relief before they go into labour.

Record-keeping and audit

Record-keeping and audit are interconnected, as the final design of the epidural record will depend on whether it is being used simply as a record of the procedure or whether it is developed as a means of gathering more extensive data about the whole of the epidural service. A detailed and accurate record of the epidural is an essential minimum requirement, but its use to collect additional material for audit of the service will depend on the resources available to the unit.

The epidural record

The record should provide accurate details of the epidural from insertion to removal. The following is a recommended format.

1. Date.
2. Time.
3. Name of person performing the epidural.
4. Grade of person performing the epidural and by whom supervised (if appropriate).
5. Consent.
6. Complications discussed.
7. Indication for epidural.
8. Technique used (for example air or saline).
9. Interspace used for epidural.
10. Depth from skin to epidural space.
11. Problems encountered during insertion of epidural needle (for example blood or dural tap).
12. Problems encountered during insertion of epidural catheter (for example blood, dural tap, paraesthesia).
13. Length of epidural catheter left in the epidural space.
14. Time taken to insert epidural.
15. Test dose:
    - drug
    - concentration
    - dose
    - time
    - blood pressure readings.
16. Prescription of local anaesthetic including dose and concentration.
17. Instructions as to whether top-ups are to be carried out by an anaesthetist or midwife.
18. Instructions for the midwife in charge of the patient – routine instructions should be part of the delivery-suite guidelines but specific instructions may need to be included.

19. Dose of top-ups and effectiveness of block – including position of patient and blood pressure.
20. Documentation of all problems encountered whilst the epidural is in place.
21. Record of the type of delivery (for example normal or forceps), comfort of the patient at delivery and any additional analgesia required.
22. Removal of epidural catheter – record whether complete.
23. Postpartum follow-up – note any problems.

The complete record should be as simple to use as possible, for example tick in a box. The chart used in the Leicester Royal Infirmary Maternity Unit is included as an example in Appendix H. This chart was developed as a national epidural chart after extensive research on and piloting by the OAA.

Audit

Audit of epidurals can encompass anything from day-to-day vigilance of work practice to a complex computerized record of epidurals performed, together with the obstetric and neonatal outcome for mother and baby.

A basic system of audit is essential to a smooth running and effective epidural service. This already exists in the form of record books kept in the maternity unit delivery suite and operating theatre. These can provide, in combination with close supervision by the consultant, a means of identifying problems and maintaining and improving the standard of the service.

For a more extensive audit, perhaps for research purposes, there are several excellent computer programmes designed to collect and collate information fed in from the epidural record. This record can be an expanded version of the example given, but too much information may be counterproductive as it becomes tedious to collect and time-consuming to feed into the computer. With faster and more user-friendly computers this should become less of a problem.

Appendix A Further reading

Aitkenhead, A. R., Smith, G. & Rowbotham, D. J. *Textbook of Anaesthesia.* Churchill Livingstone, 2006.

Baker, P. N. & Luesley, D. *Obstetrics and Gynaecology: An Evidence Based Text for MRCOG.* Taylor & Francis, 2006.

Chestnut, D. H. *Obstetric Anaesthesia: Principles and Practice,* 3rd edn. Mosby, 1999.

Collis, R., Urquhart, J. & Platt, F. eds. *Textbook of Obstetric Anaesthesia.* Greenwich Medical Media Ltd, 2002.

Gambling, D. R. & Douglas, M. J. *Obstetric Anesthesia and Uncommon Disorders.* Saunders (W. B.) Co Ltd, 1998.

Holdcroft, A. & Thomas, T. *Principles and Practice of Obstetric Anaesthesia and Analgesia.* Blackwell Science, 1999.

Nelson-Piercy, C. *Handbook of Obstetric Medicine.* Taylor & Francis, 2006.

Norman, J. & Greer, I. *Preterm Labour: Managing Risk in Clinical Practice.* Cambridge University Press, 2005.

Reynolds, F. *Regional Analgesia in Obstetrics: A Millennium Update.* Springer-Verlag London Ltd, 2000.

Yentis, S., May, A. & Malhotra, S. *Analgesia, Anaesthesia, and Pregnancy: A Practical Guide.* Cambridge University Press, 2007.

Appendix B Useful websites

National Institute for Health and Clinical Excellence, www.nice.org.uk
The Confidential Enquiry into Maternal and Child Health, www.cemach.org.uk
Obstetric Anaesthesia Association, www.oaa-anaes.ac.uk
Nursing and Midwifery Council, www.nmc-uk.org
Royal College of Midwives, www.rcm.org.uk
Royal College of Anaesthetists, www.rcoa.ac.uk
Association of Anaesthetists of Great Britain and Ireland, www.aagbi.org.uk
National Childbirth Trust, www.nct.org.uk
The Resuscitation Council (UK), www.resus.org.uk
UK Department of Health, www.dh.gov.uk

Appendix C Pain relief in labour

This booklet will give you some idea about the pain of labour and what can be done to relieve it. You will need further information from those who are looking after you about the types of pain relief available at your own hospital. We hope that if you know what to expect and, with good pain relief if need be, you will find the birth of your baby can be a satisfying experience.

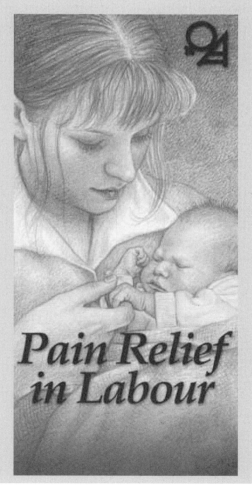

What will labour feel like?

Towards the end of pregnancy you may notice your uterus tightening from time to time. When labour starts these tightenings become regular and much stronger. This may cause pain that at first feels like strong period pain but usually gets more severe as labour progresses. The amount of pain varies. Your first labour is usually the longest and hardest. Sometimes it is necessary to start labour artificially or to stimulate it if progress is slow, and this may make it more painful. Over 90% of women find they need some sort of pain relief.

Preparing for labour

It is helpful to attend antenatal classes run by midwives who know about the hospital where you are booked. They can teach you about pregnancy and labour and caring for your baby. They will tell you what to expect when you go into hospital, what procedures may be needed and the reasons for them. Understanding what may happen during labour will make you feel less anxious. It is also helpful to visit the hospital where you plan to have your baby. All this will help you to relax and cope better.

During pregnancy physiotherapists or midwives will teach you control of breathing and ways of helping you to cope with contractions. They will also teach you correct ways of moving and good positions for working and how to relax in order to minimise problems with your joints and back, during and after your pregnancy.

At these classes you can also learn about the types of pain relief that are in use. Ask to see an anaesthetist if you want further advice about certain types of pain relief and whether they may be suitable for you. Anaesthetists are the doctors who provide epidurals, and who can also advise you about other types of pain relief. In some hospitals they give regular talks on pain relief to expectant mothers and their partners.

What methods of pain relief are available?

There are several ways of helping you cope with pain. A supportive companion is invaluable. Relaxation is important and moving around sometimes helps. Bathing in warm water and massage, particularly having your back rubbed, can help you relax and ease some pains away. Music can be helpful.

It is difficult for you to know beforehand what sort of pain relief will be best for you. The midwife who is with you in labour is the best person to advise you. Here are some of the facts about the main methods of pain relief that you may be offered.

Alternative methods

There are several ways of helping you to cope with pain, especially in early labour. Your companion can help with some of them. Although the amount of actual pain relief they produce is uncertain some people find them very helpful. You can ask whether any of these methods are used in your hospital.

- Aromatherapy
- Hypnosis
- Homeopathy
- Herbalism
- Reflexology
- Acupuncture.

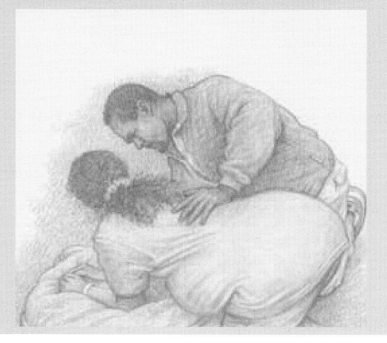

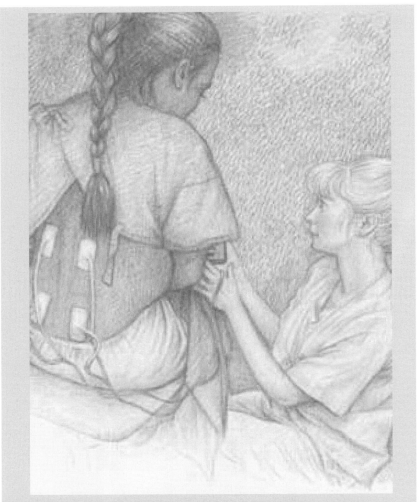

Transcutaneous electrical nerve stimulation (TENS)

- A gentle electrical current is passed through four flat pads stuck to your back. This creates a tingling feeling. You can control the strength of the current yourself.
- It is sometimes helpful at the beginning of labour, particularly for backache. If you hire one you can start it at home. Some hospitals will also lend them out.
- It has no known harmful effects on your baby.

While you may manage your labour with only the help of TENS, it is more likely that you will require some other sort of pain relief in the later stages.

Entonox

*(50% nitrous oxide and oxygen, sometimes known as **gas**)*

- You breathe this through a mask or mouthpiece.
- It is simple and quick to act, and wears off in minutes.
- It sometimes makes you feel light-headed or a little sick for a short time.
- It does not harm your baby and it gives you extra oxygen, which may be beneficial for you and your baby.
- It will not take the pain away completely but it may help.
- It can be used at any time during labour.

You, yourself, control the amount of gas you use, ***but to get the best effect timing is important.*** You should start breathing the gas as soon as you feel a contraction coming on so that you will get the full effect when the pain is at its worst. You should not use it between contractions or for long periods as this can make you feel dizzy and tingly. In some hospitals other substances may be added to the gas to make it more effective, but these may make you more sleepy.

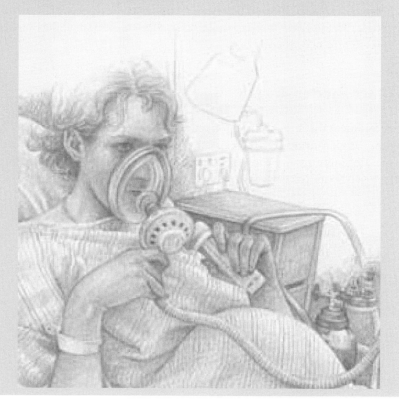

Pethidine

- Usually given by injection, into a muscle, by midwives.
- It may make you drowsy, but it may also make you less worried by the pain.
- It may make you feel sick, but you should be given something else to reduce this effect.
- It may make your baby drowsy, but an antidote can be given by injection after birth. If pethidine is given *only* shortly before delivery, the effect on your baby is very slight.
- It delays stomach emptying which might be a hazard if a general anaesthetic is needed. You should not eat or use the birthing pool if you have had pethidine.
- It may delay the establishment of breast-feeding.
- It has less effect on pain than Entonox.

Though pethidine has less effect on pain than gas, many mothers find it makes them more relaxed and able to cope with pain, though some find it disappointing.

It can also be given directly into a vein for a faster effect, and some hospitals use a machine (called Patient controlled analgesia, PCA) which allows you to press a button to give yourself measured small doses when you feel you need them.

Other injected drugs

Pethidine is the drug licensed for use by midwives, although a number of other similar drugs have been used to relieve labour pain. Those worth mentioning are diamorphine, fentanyl and meptazinol, which some units feel give better pain relief. They act in a similar way to pethidine.

Epidurals

- Given into a very small tube in your back.
- Most complicated method, performed by an anaesthetist.
- Little effect on your baby.
- A small risk of headache.
- May cause a drop in blood pressure.
- Most effective method of pain relief.

Who should have an epidural?

Most people can have an epidural, but certain complications of pregnancy and bleeding disorders may make it unsuitable. If you have a complicated or long labour your midwife or obstetrician may recommend that you have one. In such circumstances it will benefit you and your baby.

What does it involve?

You will first need a drip, that is fluid running in to a vein in your arm. This is often necessary in labour for other reasons. You will be asked to curl up on your side or sit bending forwards. Your back will be cleaned and a little injection of local anaesthetic given into the skin, so putting in the epidural should hardly hurt. A small tube is put into your back near the nerves carrying pain from the uterus. Care is needed to avoid puncturing the bag of fluid that surrounds the spinal cord, as this may give you a headache afterwards. It is therefore important to keep still while the anaesthetist is putting in the epidural, but after the tube is in place you will be free to move.

Once the tube is in place, pain-relieving drugs can be given as often as is necessary, or continuously by a pump. While the epidural is taking effect, the midwife will take your blood pressure regularly. The anaesthetist and your midwife will also check that the epidural is working properly. It usually takes about 20 minutes to work, but occasionally it doesn't work well at first, and some adjustment is needed.

What are the effects?

- Nowadays it is usually possible to provide pain relief without numbness or heavy legs, in other words a 'mobile epidural'.
- An epidural should not make you feel drowsy or sick, nor does it normally delay stomach emptying.
- Occasionally it drops your blood pressure, which is why you have the drip.
- An epidural may prolong the second stage of labour and reduce the urge to bear down. Occasionally this may result in you having an instrumental delivery, but you are still more likely to have a normal delivery than any other type of delivery.
- It removes much of the stress of labour, which is good for the baby.
- Breast-feeding is not impaired, in fact it is often helped.

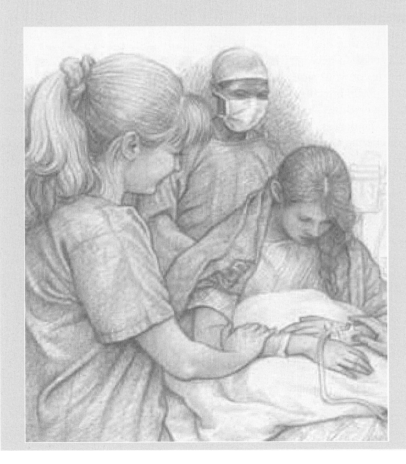

- In this country as a whole, there is less than a one in 100 chance of your getting a severe headache after an epidural, but hospitals vary in their headache rate so you might enquire about this. If you develop a headache afterwards, it can be treated. A leaflet is available, produced by the Royal College and the Association of Anaesthetists, *Headaches after Spinal and Epidural Anaesthesia*, which gives further information.
- Backache is common during pregnancy and often continues afterwards when you are looking after your baby. There is now good evidence that epidurals do **not** cause long-term backache, though you may feel local tenderness for a day or two afterwards.
- About one in 2000 mothers gets a feeling of tingling or pins and needles down one leg after having a baby. Such problems are more likely to result from childbirth itself than from an epidural. Other more serious problems happen even more rarely.

What if you need an operation?

If you should need any operation such as caesarean section or forceps delivery, you may not need a general anaesthetic, as the epidural can often be used instead. A stronger local anaesthetic and other pain-relieving drugs can be injected into your epidural tube to provide an adequate anaesthetic for your operation. This is safer for you and the baby.

What about spinals?

Epidurals are rather slow to act, particularly in late labour. If the pain-killing drugs are put directly into the bag of fluid surrounding the nerves in your back, they work much faster. This is called a spinal. A much smaller needle is used for a spinal than for an epidural, so the risk of headache is small. In some hospitals spinals, or a combination of spinals and epidurals, are used for pain relief in labour and spinal anaesthesia is commonly used for caesarean section.

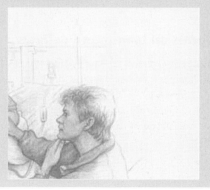

Bibliography

Relative merits of different types of pain relief

Chamberlain G, Wraight A, Steer P, eds. *Pain and its relief in childbirth: The results of a national survey conducted by the National Birthday Trust.* Edinburgh, Churchill Livingstone, 1993:pp49–67.

Melzack R, Taenzer P, Feldman P, Kinch RA. Labour is still painful after prepared childbirth training. *Can Med Assoc J* 1981;**125**:357–63.

Keirse MJNC, Enkin M, Lumley J. Support from caregivers during childbirth. In: *The Cochrane Pregnancy and Childbirth Database. The Cochrane Collaboration and Update Software*, 1995; issue 1.

Ranta P, Jouppila P, Spalding M, Kangas-Saarela T, Hollmén A, Jouppila R. Parturients' assessment of water blocks, pethidine, nitrous oxide, paracervical and epidural blocks in labour. *International Journal of Obstetric Anesthesia* 1994;**3**:193–8.

Carrol D, Tramer M, McQuay H et al. Transcutaneous electrical nerve stimulation in labour pain: a systemic review. *Br J Obstet Gynaecol* 1997;**104**:169–75.

Nikkola EM, Ulla UE, Penti OK et al. Intravenous fentanyl PCA during labour. *Can J Anaesth* 1997;**44**:1248–55.

Holdcroft A, Morgan M. An assessment of the analgesic effect in labour of pethidine and 50 per cent nitrous oxide in oxygen (Entonox). *J Obstet Gynaecol Br Commonw* 1974;**81**:603–7.

Ross JA, Tunstall ME, Campbell D et al. The use of 0.25% isoflurane premixed in 50% nitrous oxide and oxygen for pain relief in labour. *Anaesthesia* 1999;**54**:1166–72.

Olofsson C, Ekblom A, Ekman-Ordeberg G, Hjelm A, Irestedt L. Lack of analgesic effect of systemically administered morphine or pethidine on labour pain. *Br J Obstet Gynaecol* 1996;**103**:968–72.

Harrison RF, Shore M, Woods T, Mathews G, Gardiner J, Unwin A. A comparative study of transcutaneous electrical nerve stimulation (TENS), Entonox, pethidine + promazine and lumbar epidural for pain relief in labour. *Acta Obstet Gynecol Scand* 1987;**66**:9–14.

Wee MYK, Hasan MA, Thomas TA, Isoflurane in labour. *Anaesthesia* 1993;**48**:369–72.

Effects of epidurals on labour and delivery

Halpern SH, Leighton BL, Ohlsson A, Barrett JFR, Rice A. Effect of epidural vs parenteral opioid analgesia on the progress of labour. (A meta-analysis of 9 randomised trials.) *JAMA* 1998;**280**:2105–10.

Zhang J, Klebanoff MA, DerSimonian R. Epidural analgesia in association with duration of labor and mode of delivery: A quantitative review. *Am J Obstet Gynecol* 1999;**180**:970–7.

Effects on the baby

Reynolds F. ed: *Effects on the baby of maternal analgesia and anaesthesia.* London, WB Saunders 1993.

Huch A, Huch R, Schneider H, Rooth G. Continuous transcutaneous monitoring of fetal oxygen tension during labour. *Br J Obstet Gynaecol* 1977;**84**(Suppl. 1):1–39.

Belfrage P, Boreus LO, Hartvig P et al. Neonatal depression after obstetrical analgesia with pethidine: the role of the injection-delivery time interval and of the plasma concentrations of pethidine and norpethidine. *Acta Obstet Gynecol Scand* 1981;**60**:43–9.

Hamza J, Benlabed M, Orhant E, Escourrou P, Curzi-Dascalova L, Gaultier C. Neonatal pattern of breathing during active and quiet sleep after maternal administration of meperidine. *Pediatr Res* 1992;**32**:412–6.

Weiner PC, Hogg MJ, Rosen M. Effects of naloxone on pethidine induced neonatal depression. *BMJ* 1977;**2**:228–31.

Crowell MK, Hill PD, Humerick SS. Relationship between obstetric analgesia and time of effective breast feeding. *Journal of Nurse-Midwifery* 1994;**39**:150–6.

Kotelko DM, Faulk DL, Rottman RL, et al. A controlled comparison of maternal analgesia: effects on neonatal nutritional sucking behavior. *Anesthesiology* 1995;**83**:A927.

Hirose M, Hara Y, Hosokawa T, Tanaka Y. The effect of postoperative analgesia with continuous epidural bupivacaine after cesarean section on the amount of breast feeding and infant weight gain. *Anesth Analg* 1996;**82**:1166–9.

Effects on the gastrointestinal tract

Petring OU, Adelhof B, Erinmadsen J, Angelo H, Jelert H. Epidural anaesthesia does not delay early postoperative gastric emptying in man. *Acta Anaesthesiol Scand* 1984;**28**:393–5.

Nimmo WS, Wilson J, Prescott LF. Narcotic analgesia and delayed gastric emptying during labour. *Lancet* 1975;i:890–3.

Incidence of complications

i. Effect on Mobility

Russell R, Reynolds F. Epidural infusion of low-dose bupivacaine and opioid in labour. Does reducing motor block increase the spontaneous delivery rate? *Anaesthesia* 1996;**51**:266–73.

Collis RE, Davies DWL, Aveling W. Randomised comparison of combined spinal-epidural with standard epidural analgesia in labour. *Lancet* 1995;**345**:1413–6.

ii. Headaches

Gleeson C, Reynolds F. Accidental dural puncture rates in UK obstetric practice. *International Journal of Obstetric Anesthesia* 1998;**67**:242–6.

Paech MJ, Godkin R, Webster S. Complications of obstetric epidural analgesia and anaesthesia: a prospective analysis of 10995 cases. *International Journal of Obstetric Anesthesia* 1998;**7**:5–11.

Royal College and Association of Anaesthetists. *Headaches after Spinal and Epidural Anaesthesia* 2003.

iii. Lack of association with backache

Russell R, Dundas R, Reynolds F. Long term backache after childbirth: prospective search for causative factors. *BMJ* 1996;**312**:1384–8.

Breen TW, Ransil BJ, Groves P, Oriol NE. Factors associated with back pain after childbirth. *Anesthesiology* 1994;**81**:29–34.

Macarthur A, Macarthur C, Weeks S. Epidural anesthesia and long term back pain after delivery: a prospective cohort study. *BMJ* 1995;**311**:1336–9.

Loughnan BA, Carli F, Romney M, Dore C, Gordon H. The influence of epidural analgesia on the development of new backache in primiparous women: report of a randomized controlled trial. *International Journal of Obstetric Anesthesia* 1997;**6**:203–4.

Neurological complications of childbirth

Holdcroft A, Gibberd FB, Hargrove RL, Hawkins DF, Dellaportas CI. Neurological complications associated with pregnancy. *Br J Anaesth* 1995;**75**:522–6.

Paech MJ, Godkin R, Webster S. Complications of obstetric epidural analgesia and anaesthesia: a prospective analysis of 10995 cases. *International Journal of Obstetric Anesthesia* 1998;**7**:5–11.

Loo CC, Dahlgren G, Irestedt L. Neurological complications in obstetric regional anaesthesia. *International Journal of Obstetric Anesthesia* 2000;**9**:99–124.

- *The information in this booklet is based on good evidence; some of the publications from which it is derived are listed.*
- *The Obstetric Anaesthetists' Association also produce a booklet for mothers on **Caesarean section: your choice of anaesthesia** and two films on a double DVD called **Coping with labour pain** and **Your anaesthetic for Caesarean section**.*
- *Both booklets may be found on the Association's website along with a number of translations.*
- *A booklet on **Headache after an epidural or spinal anaesthetic** has been jointly produced by the Royal College of Anaesthetists and the Association of Anaesthetists and can be downloaded from **www.youranaesthetic.info**.*

This booklet was written by the Information for Mothers Subcommittee of the Obstetric Anaesthetists' Association.

Dr Michael Wee (chairman), Prof Felicity Reynolds,
Dr Michael Bryson, Mrs Carol Bates (RCM representative),
Mrs Cathy Groeger (AIMS representative),

Mrs Christina Campbell (Consumer representative),
Mrs Shaheen Chaudry, Dr Michael Kinsella,
Dr Geraldine O'Sullivan, Dr Roshan Fernando.

Further copies of both OAA booklets and the double DVD may be obtained from the Secretariat of the Obstetric Anaesthetists' Association

OAA Secretariat
PO Box 3219, Barnes
London SW13 9XR
Tel: +44 (0)20 8741 1311
Fax: +44 (0)20 8741 0611
Email: secretariat@oaa-anaes.ac.uk
Web: www.oaa-anaes.ac.uk

2nd Edition Revised October 2003, reprinted October 2005

Appendix D Caesarean section: your choice of anaesthesia

About one in five babies is born by **caesarean section** and two thirds of these are unexpected; so you may like to glance at this booklet, even if you do not expect to have a caesarean yourself.

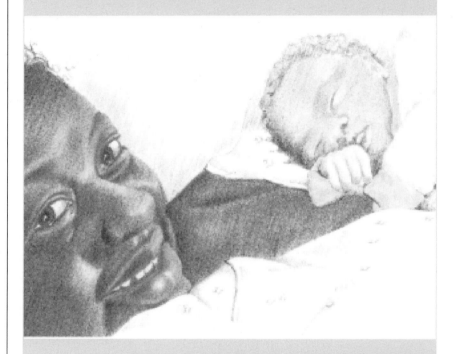

Having a baby is an unforgettable experience

A caesarean section can be just as satisfying as a vaginal delivery, and if it turns out you need a caesarean section, you should not feel this is in any sense a failure. The most important thing is that you and your baby are safe. A caesarean section may be the best way to ensure this.

There are several types of anaesthesia for caesarean section. This booklet explains the various choices. You can discuss the choice of anaesthetic with your anaesthetist. Obstetric anaesthetists are doctors who specialise in the anaesthetic care and welfare of pregnant women and their babies.

Your caesarean section may be planned in advance; this is called an *elective caesarean section*. This may be advisable if there is an increased chance of complications developing during a vaginal delivery. One example might be if your baby is in an unusual position in the later stages of pregnancy.

In some cases, caesarean section may be recommended in a hurry, usually when you are already in labour. This is an *emergency caesarean section*. This may be recommended because of poor progress in labour; because the baby's condition is deteriorating or a combination of the two.

Your obstetrician will discuss with you the reasons for your caesarean section and obtain consent for the operation.

Types of anaesthesia

There are two main types; you can be either awake or asleep. Most caesareans are done under regional anaesthesia, when you are awake but sensation from the lower body is numbed. It is usually safer for mother and baby and allows both you and your partner to experience the birth together.

There are three types of regional anaesthesia:

1. Spinal – the most commonly used method. It may be used in planned or emergency caesarean section. The nerves and spinal cord that carry feelings from your lower body (and messages to make your muscles move) are contained in a bag of fluid inside your backbone. Local anaesthetic is put inside this bag of fluid, using a very fine needle. A spinal works fast with a small dose of anaesthetic.

REGIONAL ANAESTHESIA

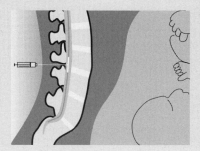

2. Epidural – A thin plastic tube or catheter is put outside the bag of fluid, near the nerves carrying pain from the uterus. An epidural is often used to treat the pain of labour using weak local anaesthetic solutions. It can be topped up if you need a caesarean section by giving a stronger local anaesthetic solution. In an epidural, a larger dose of local anaesthetic is necessary than with a spinal, and it takes longer to work. Your epidural can be topped up if needed.

3. Combined spinal-epidural or CSE – a combination of the two. The spinal can be used for the caesarean section. The epidural can be used to give more anaesthetic if required, and to give pain-relieving drugs after the operation.

General anaesthesia – If you have a general anaesthetic you will be asleep for the caesarean section. General anaesthesia is used less often nowadays. It may be needed for some emergencies; if there is a reason why regional anaesthesia is unsuitable or if you prefer to be asleep.

The pros and cons of each are described later in this booklet. First it is useful to know what happens when a caesarean section is planned, and a date given for your operation.

Pre-operative assessment

Normally you will visit the hospital before you come in for your operation. The midwife will see you and take some blood from you for tests before the operation. She will also explain what to expect. Most women go home after the assessment and come back to hospital on the day of the operation, but you may need to stay in the night before. You may be given tablets to reduce the acid in your stomach and prevent sickness; you need to take one the night before the operation and one on the morning itself. This will be explained to you.

The anaesthetist's visit

You should be seen by an anaesthetist before your caesarean section. The anaesthetist will review your medical history and any previous anaesthetics. You may need an examination or further tests. The anaesthetist will also discuss the anaesthetic choices with you and answer your questions.

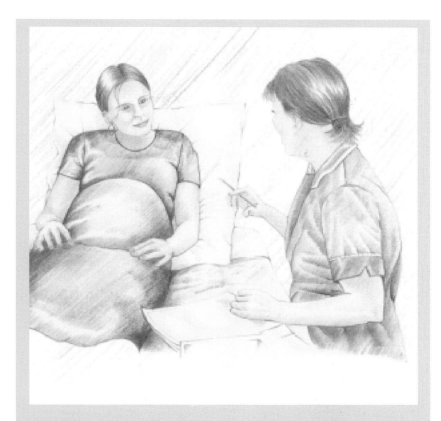

On the day

The midwife will confirm the time of your operation and check that you have taken your tablets. Your bikini line may need to be shaved. You will have a name band on your wrist or ankle. The midwife may help you to put on special tight stockings (called TED stockings) to prevent clots forming in your legs. You will be given a theatre gown to put on. Your birthing partner can accompany you and the midwife to the operating theatre. Special theatre clothes will be provided.

In theatre, equipment will be attached to measure your blood pressure, heart rate, and the amount of oxygen in your blood, quite painlessly. Using a local anaesthetic to numb your skin, the anaesthetist will set up a drip to give you fluid through your veins. Then the anaesthetic will be started.

What will happen if you have regional anaesthesia?

You'll be asked either to sit or to lie on your side, curling your back. The anaesthetist will paint your back with sterilising solution, which feels cold. He or she will then find a suitable point in the middle of the lower back and will give you a little local anaesthetic injection to numb the skin. This sometimes stings for a moment.

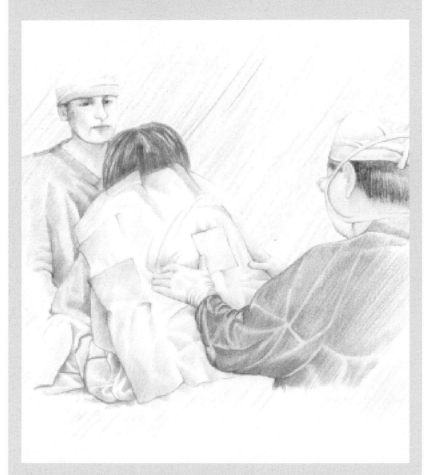

Then for a spinal, a fine spinal needle is put into your back; this is not usually painful. Sometimes, you might feel a tingling going down one leg as the needle goes in, like a small electric shock. You should mention this, but it is important that you keep still while the spinal is being put in. When the needle is in the right position, local anaesthetic and a pain-relieving drug will be injected and the needle removed. It usually takes just a few minutes, but if it is difficult to place the needle, it may take longer.

For an epidural, a larger needle is needed to allow the epidural catheter to be threaded down it into the epidural space. As with a spinal, this sometimes causes a tingling feeling or small electric shock down your leg. It is important to keep still while the anaesthetist is putting in the epidural, but once the catheter is in place, the needle is removed and you don't have to keep still.

If you already have an epidural catheter for pain relief in labour, then all the anaesthetist has to do is put a stronger dose of local anaesthetic down the catheter, which should work well for a caesarean section. If the caesarean section is very urgent, it may be decided that there is not enough time for the epidural to be extended, so a different anaesthetic may be recommended.

You will know when the spinal or epidural is working because your legs begin to feel heavy and warm. They may also start to tingle. Numbness will spread gradually up your body. The anaesthetist will check how far the block has spread to make sure that you are ready for the operation. It is sometimes necessary to change your position to make sure the anaesthetic is working well. Your blood pressure will be taken frequently.

While the anaesthetic is taking effect, a midwife will insert a tube (a urinary catheter) into your bladder to keep it empty during the operation. This should not be uncomfortable. The tube may be left in place until the next morning, so you won't need to worry about being able to pass water.

For the operation, you will be placed on your back with a tilt towards the left side. If you feel sick at any time, you should mention this to the anaesthetist. It is often caused by a drop in blood pressure. The anaesthetist will give you appropriate treatment to help you.

Until the baby is born, you may be given oxygen through a transparent plastic mask to make sure the baby has plenty of oxygen before the birth.

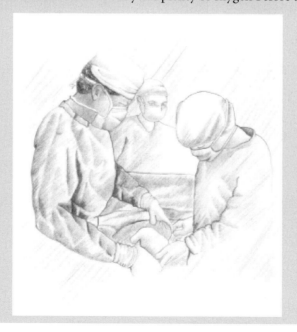

The operation

A screen separates you and your birthing partner from the operation site. The anaesthetist will stay with you all the time. You may hear a lot of preparation in the background. This is because the obstetricians work with a team of midwives and theatre staff.

Your skin is usually cut slightly below the bikini line. Once the operation is under way, you may feel pulling and pressure, but you should not feel pain. Some women have described it as feeling like 'someone doing the washing-up inside my tummy'. The anaesthetist will assess you throughout the procedure and can give you more pain relief if required. Whilst it is unusual, occasionally it may be necessary to give you a general anaesthetic.

From the start it takes about ten minutes before the delivery. Immediately after the birth, the midwife quickly dries and examines your baby. A paediatrician may do this with the midwife. After this, you and your partner will be able to cuddle your baby.

After the birth, a drug called Syntocinon is put into your drip to help tighten your uterus and deliver your placenta. An antibiotic will also be put into the drip to reduce the risk of wound infection. The obstetrician will take about another half-hour to complete the operation. Afterwards, you may be given a suppository in your back passage to relieve pain when the anaesthetic wears off.

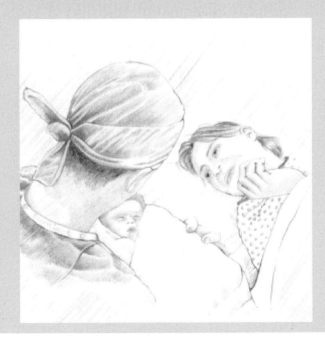

When the operation is over

You should be helped to sit up slightly, and then taken to the recovery room where you will be under observation for a while. Your partner and baby can usually be with you. Your baby will be weighed and then you can begin breast feeding if you like. In the recovery room, your anaesthetic will gradually wear off and you may feel a tingling sensation in your legs. Within a couple of hours you'll be able to move them again. The pain relieving drugs given with your spinal or epidural should continue to give you pain relief for a few hours. When you need more pain relief, ask the midwife.

What will happen with general anaesthesia?

You will be given an antacid to drink and a urinary catheter will be inserted before your general anaesthetic. The anaesthetist will give you oxygen to breathe through a facemask for a few minutes. Once the obstetrician and all the team are assembled, the anaesthetist will give the anaesthetic in your drip to send you to sleep. Just before you go off to sleep, the anaesthetist's assistant will press lightly on your neck. This is to prevent stomach fluid getting into your lungs. The anaesthetic works very quickly.

When you are asleep, a tube is put into your windpipe to prevent stomach contents from entering your lungs and to allow a machine to breathe for you. The anaesthetist will continue the anaesthetic to keep you asleep and allow the obstetrician to deliver your baby safely. But you won't know anything about all this.

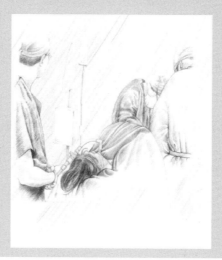

When you wake up, your throat may feel uncomfortable from the tube, and you may feel sore from the operation. You may also feel sleepy and perhaps nauseated, for a while. But you should soon be back to normal. You will be wheeled to the recovery area where you will meet up with your baby and partner. You may be given a patient controlled analgesia (PCA) machine, which provides you with pain relief at a press of a button whenever you need it. If not, ask the midwife when you need more painkillers.

Some reasons why you may need general anaesthesia:

- In certain conditions when the blood cannot clot properly, regional anaesthesia is best avoided.
- There may not be enough time for regional anaesthesia to work.
- A very abnormal back may make regional anaesthesia difficult or impossible.
- Occasionally, spinal or epidural anaesthesia does not work well.

Pain relief after the operation

There are several ways to give you pain relief after caesarean section:

- Regional: you can be given a long acting pain killer with the spinal or epidural.
- Epidural: in some hospitals the epidural catheter is left in for later use.
- Suppositories are often given at the end of the operation.
- Injection into a muscle of morphine or similar painkiller, by a midwife.
- Into a drip: (morphine or similar drug) you can control the amount yourself. This is called patient-controlled analgesia or PCA.
- By mouth: a midwife can give you tablets such as Voltarol or paracetamol.

Advantages of regional compared with general anaesthesia

- Spinals and epidurals are usually safer for you and your baby.
- They enable you and your partner to share in the birth.
- You won't be sleepy afterwards.
- They allow earlier feeding and contact with your baby.
- You will have good pain relief afterwards.
- Your baby will be born more alert.

Disadvantages of regional compared with general anaesthesia

- Spinals and epidurals can lower the blood pressure, though this is easily treated.
- In general, they may take longer to set up than a general anaesthetic.
- Occasionally, they may make you feel shaky.
- Rarely, they don't work perfectly; so a general anaesthetic may be necessary.

Also they may cause:

- Tingling down one leg, more with spinals. (In about one in ten thousand spinals, this may last several weeks or months).
- Itching during the operation and afterwards, but this can be treated.
- Severe headache, in fewer than one in a hundred women. This can be treated.
- Local tenderness in your back for a few days. This is not unusual.

Spinals and epidurals do not cause chronic backache

Unfortunately backache is very common after childbirth, particularly among women who have suffered with it before or during pregnancy, but spinals and epidurals do not make it more so.

Having a baby by caesarean section is safe and can be a very rewarding experience. Many women choose to be awake for the procedure. Others may need to be asleep for the reasons discussed above. We hope that this booklet will enable you to make an informed choice for your caesarean section.

Bibliography

Caesarean section with regional anaesthesia

Kennedy BW, Thorp JM, Fitch W, Millar K. The theatre environment and the awake patient. *J Obstet Gynaecol* 1992;12:407–411.

Ying LC, Levy V, Shan CO, Hung TW, Wah WK. A qualitative study of the perceptions of Hong Kong Chinese women during caesarean section under regional anaesthesia. *Midwifery* 2001;17:115–22.

Relative merits of different types of anaesthesia

Shibli KU, Russell IF. A survey of anaesthetic techniques used for caesarean section in the UK in 1997. *Int J Obstet Anesth* 2000; 9: 160–7.

Riley ET, Cohen SE, Macario A, Desai JB, Ratner EF. Spinal versus epidural anesthesia for cesarean section: a comparison of time efficiency, costs, charges, and complications. *Anesth Analg* 1995;80:709–12.

Davies SJ, Paech MJ, Welch H, Evans SF, Pavy TJG. Maternal experience during epidural or combined spinalepidural anesthesia for cesarean section: a prospective randomized trial. *Anesth Analg* 1997;85:607–13.

Morgan PJ, Halpern S, Lam-McCulloch J. Comparison of maternal satisfaction between epidural and spinal anesthesia for elective Cesarean section. *Can J Anaesth* 2000;47:956–61.

Effects of different types of anaesthesia on the baby

Marx GF, Luykx WM, Cohen S. Fetal-neonatal status following caesarean section for fetal distress. *Br J Anaesth* 1984; 56: 1009–1013.

Abboud TK, Nagappala S, Murakawa K et al. Comparison of the effects of general and regional anesthesia for cesarean section on neonatal neurologic and adaptive capacity scores. *Anesth Anal* 1985; 64: 996–1000.

Ong BY, Cohen MM, Palahniuk RJ. Anesthesia for Cesarean section – effects on neonates. *Anesth Analg* 1989;68:270–5.

Evans CM, Murphy JF, Gray OL, Rosen M. Epidural versus general anaesthesia for elective Caesarean section. Effect on Apgar score and acid-base status of the newborn. *Anaesthesia* 1989;44:778–82.

Mahajan J, Mahajan RP, Singh MM, Anand NK. Anaesthetic technique for elective caesarean section and neurobehavioural status of newborns. *Int J Obstet Anesth* 1993;2:89–93.

Hodgson CA, Wauchob TD. A comparison of spinal and general anaesthesia for elective caesarean section: Effect on neonatal condition at birth. *Int J Obstet Anesth* 1994; 3: 25–30.

Ratcliffe FM, Evans JM. Neonatal wellbeing after elective caesarean delivery with general, spinal and epidural anaesthesia. *Eur J Anesthesiol* 1998; 10: 175–81.

Kolatat T, Somboonnanonda A, Lertakyamanee J, Chinachot T, Tritrakarn T, Muangkasem J. Effects of general and regional anesthesia on the neonate (a prospective, randomized trial). *J Med Assoc Thailand* 1999; 82: 40–5.

Dick W, Traub E, Kraus H, Tollner U, Burghard R, Muck J. General anaesthesia versus epidural anaesthesia for primary Caesarean section: A comparative study. *Eur J Anaesthesiol* 1992;9:15–21.

Pain relief after caesarean section

Morrison J D, McGrady E M. Postoperative pain relief. Chapter in: Reynolds F (ed). *Regional analgesia in obstetrics: a millenium update*. London: Springer-Verlag, 2000.

Graham D, Russell IF. A double-blind assessment of the analgesic sparing effect of intrathecal diamorphine (0.3 mg) with spinal anaesthesia for elective caesarean section. *Int J Obstet Anesth* 1997; 6: 224–30.

Husaini SW, Russell IF. Intrathecal diamorphine compared with morphine for postoperative analgesia after Caesarean section under spinal anaesthesia. *Br J Anaesth* 1998;81:135–9.

Van de Velde M. What is the best way to provide postoperative pain therapy after caesarean section? *Curr Opinion Anaesthesiol* 2000;13:267–70.

Incidence of complications

Headache:

Reynolds F. Dural puncture and headache. Chapter in: Reynolds F (ed). *Regional analgesia in obstetrics: a millenium update*. London: Springer-Verlag, 2000.

Backache:

Russell R, Reynolds F. Back pain, pregnancy and childbirth. [Editorial]. *Br Med J* 1997;314:1062–3.

Nerve damage:

Holdcroft A, Gibberd FB, Hargrove RL, Hawkins DF, Dellaportas CI. Neurological complications associated with pregnancy. *Br J Anaesth* 1995;75:522–6.

Loo CC, Dahlgren G, Irestedt L. Neurological complications in obstetric regional anaesthesia. *Int J Obstet Anesth* 2000; 9: 99–124.

Paech MJ, Godkin R, Webster S. Complications of obstetric epidural analgesia and anaesthesia: a prospective analysis of 10,995 cases. *Int J Obstet Anesth* 1998;7:5–11.

Further reading

Reynolds F (ed). *Regional analgesia in obstetrics: a millennium update*. London: Springer-Verlag, 2000.

Russell R, Porter J, Scrutton M. *Pain Relief in Labour*. Ed F Reynolds. London: BMJ Publishing, 1997.

Acknowledgements

The information in this booklet is based on good evidence; some of the publications from which it is derived are listed.

The booklet was written by the Information for Mothers Subcommittee of the Obstetric Anaesthetists Association.

Dr Michael Wee (chairman), Prof Felicity Reynolds, Dr Michael Bryson, Mrs Carol Bates (RCM representative), Mrs Cathy Groeger (AIMS representative), Mrs Christina Campbell (Consumer representative), Mrs Shaheen Chaudhry (Consumer representative), Dr Michael Kinsella, Dr Geraldine O'Sullivan, Dr Roshan Fernando.

Further information on anaesthesia can be obtained from www.youranaesthetic.info.

- A video produced by the Obstetric Anaesthetists Association entitled 'Your anaesthetic for Caesarean section' has been produced to accompany this booklet.
- Further copies of the booklet and the Caesarean section video can be obtained from the Secretariat of the Obstetric Anaesthetists' Association. Website: www.oaa-anaes.ac.uk.

OAA Secretariat
PO Box 3219, Barnes
London SW13 9XR
Tel: +44 (0)20 8741 1311
Fax: +44 (0)20 8741 0611
E-mail: secretariat@oaa-anaes.ac.uk
First Edition March 2003

Appendix E Epidural information card

EPIDURAL INFORMATION CARD
Epidurals in labour – what you need to know

(This card is intended as a summary only. Please discuss any issues with your anaesthetist)

Setting up your epidural
- You would need to have a drip.
- While the epidural is being put in it is absolutely essential that you keep still and let the anaesthetist know if you are having a contraction.
- Usually takes 20 minutes to set up and 20 minutes to work.
- Some epidurals do not work fully and need to be adjusted or replaced.

Advantages of an epidural
- Usually provides excellent pain relief.
- Can be adjusted to allow you to move around the bed and push the baby out.
- Can be topped up for caesarean section if required.
- In general epidurals do not affect your baby.
- The low-dose or mobile epidurals do not seem to delay labour.

Possible problems with your epidural
- Repeated top-ups with stronger solutions may prolong your labour and cause your legs to become heavy.
- Mild itching is very common after epidural top-ups but rarely causes a problem.
- The epidural site may be tender but usually only for a few days. Backache is NOT caused by epidurals but is common after any pregnancy.

PTO: Important side-effects are on the other side of this card.

EPIDURAL INFORMATION CARD
Side-effect/problems of epidurals

Side-effect	How often?	How common?
Partially working or not working at all	1:100 or 1 in family	Common
Bad headache	1:200 or 1 in a street	Uncommon
Drop in blood pressure	1:1000 or 1 person in a small village	Rare
Nerve damage – numb patch on thigh or weak leg: (1) temporary (a few weeks to months) (2) permanent	 1:1000–2000 or 1 person in an inner city housing estate 1:13 000 or 1 person in a small town	 Rare Very rare
Paralysis	1:1000 000 or 1 person in a city	Very, very rare

PTO: For general information about epidurals during labour

Appendix F Suggested list of trolley contents

Epidural Trolley Checklist

Top of trolley

Sterile gloves (including latex free – Dermaprene)
Anaesthetic charts
Masks
Epidural pack (sterile)
Patient gown
Chlorhexidine spray

1st drawer

Saline 10 ml
2% Lidocaine (Lignocaine) 5 ml
2% Lidocaine (Lignocaine) 20 ml
0.5% Bupivacaine/Levobupivacaine (Chirocaine) 10 ml
0.25% Bupivacaine/Levobupivacaine (Chirocaine) 10 ml
Ephedrine 30 mg/1 ml
Epinephrine (Adrenaline) 1 mg/1 ml
Ethyl Chloride spray
Roll of Tape

2nd drawer

Needles: 25G (orange), 22G (blue), 18G (green), 17G (white), filter,
  drawing-up
Syringes: 1 ml, 2 ml, 5 ml, 10 ml, 20 ml
Plasters
Bungs
Disposable scalpel size 11
Multi-Adaptor for:
Monovette Blood Bottles (few of each, no more)

3rd drawer

Syringe labels: Lidocaine (Lignocaine), Bupivacaine, Ephedrine
Additive labels (yellow)
Spinal needles (24G Sprotte): 90 mm, 120 mm *only*
Tuohy needles (winged): 150 mm
Individual epidural filters, catheters, LOR syringes
Cannulae: 16G(grey) with one of each of 18G(green), 20G(pink), 25G(yellow)
Epidural mini packs

4th drawer

Mefix: 1 box of narrow, 1 box of wide
One way valves
Line splitters: doubles and trebles
IV extension lines

5th drawer

Hartmann's solution 1000 ml $\times$ 4
Gelatin (Gelofusine/Haemaccel) 500 ml $\times$ 2
Saline 0.9% 1000 ml $\times$ 2

Appendix G Dermatome chart

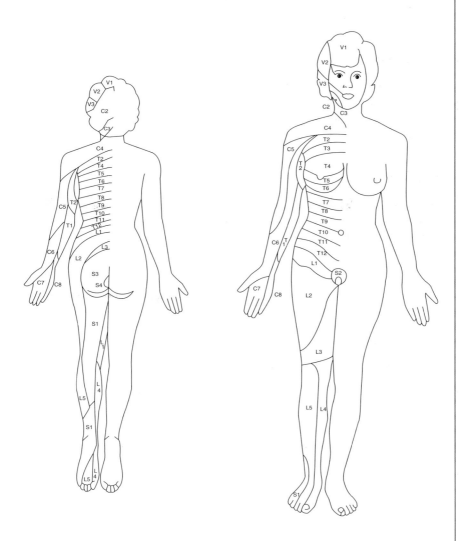

The National Maternity Record (PILOT)	**Epidural Analgesia Chart for Labour**		
Date	Previous epidural(s)	N ☐	Y ☐
	Previous LSCS(s)	N ☐	Y ☐
	Medical problem(s)	N ☐	Y ☐
	Normal back	Y ☐	N ☐
	Fetal concern(s)	N ☐	Y ☐
	Previous anaesthetic problem(s)	N ☐	Y ☐
	Potential difficult airway	N ☐	Y ☐

Height (cm)	Weight (kg)	Allergies
Relevant investigations		
Parity	Cervical dilatation (cm)	
Analgesia already used		

INFORMATION FOR WOMEN PRIOR TO ACCEPTANCE OF PROFESSIONAL ADVICE (consent)

Consent taken		Verbal ☐		Written ☐	See pg. 9 National Maternity Record
Name	PRINT			Signature	
Doctor/Midwife					
Patient/Witness					
Midwife present	Y ☐	N ☐	Partner present	Y ☐	N ☐
Warnings of:		Headache ☐	Hypotension ☐	Technique failure ☐	
			Dural puncture ☐	Pruritus ☐	

INFORMATION RECORDED WHILST SITING EPIDURAL CATHETER

Anaesthetist	Cons ☐	Ass Spec ☐	SG ☐	SpR (yr) ☐	SHO (yr) ☐	Other
				Permanent ☐	Locum ☐	
Name	PRINT				Signature	
2nd Anaesthetist	Cons ☐	Ass Spec ☐	SG ☐	SpR (yr) ☐	SHO (yr) ☐	Other
Name	PRINT				Signature	

TECHNIQUE (tick one or more in each line)

Asepsis	Gown ☐	Gloves ☐	Mask ☐	Skin preparation	
Block	Lumbar epidural ☐	Spinal ☐	CSE ☐	Other	
Position	Lateral ☐	Sitting ☐		Other	
Needle type	Tuohy ___G ☐	Spinal ___G ☐	Pencil point type ☐	Other	
Space(s) used	L4/5 ☐	L3/4 ☐	L2/3 ☐	L1/2 ☐	Other
Approach	Midline ☐	Paramedian ☐			
No. of reasonable attempts	1 ☐	2 ☐	3 ☐	>3 ☐	
Loss of resistance	Air ☐	Saline ☐		Other	
Depth	Of space (cm) [____]		Length of catheter in space (cm) [____]		

TECHNICAL PROBLEMS

Insertion difficulties	None ☐	Obese ☐	Movement ☐	Bone ☐	Other	
Blood in catheter	N ☐	Y ☐	Flushed clear:		N ☐	Y ☐
			Re-sited:		N ☐	Y ☐
Dural tap	N ☐	Y ☐	With needle ☐	With catheter ☐	Which space [____]	
Parasthesia on insertion	N ☐	Y ☐	When [____]		Distribution [____]	
Comments						

FOLLOW-UP AFTER ANAESTHETIC INTERVENTION

Date of follow-up	Dr's Signature	PRINT NAME

Anaesthetic intervention (Tick one or more of these boxes)

Ep= Epidural   Sp= Spinal   CSE= Combined Spinal-Epidural   GA= General Anaesthetic   RB= Regional Block

		Ep ☐	Sp ☐	CSE ☐	GA ☐
	Ep+Sp ☐	Ep+CSE ☐	Ep+GA ☐	Sp+GA ☐	CSE+GA ☐
				Ep+CSE+GA ☐	Ep+Sp+GA ☐
Attempted RB failed ☐		Attempted RB baby delivered ☐			
Other ☐					

Mode of delivery   NSVD ☐   Vaginal assisted ☐   EmLSCS ☐   EILSCS ☐

Pain relief	in labour	Good ☐	Moderate ☐	Poor ☐
Pain relief	for delivery	Good ☐	Moderate ☐	Poor ☐
Maternal view	of pain relief in labour	Very satisfied ☐	Satisfied ☐	Dissatisfied ☐
		Delay in establishing pain relief ☐	Missed segments ☐	Unilateral block ☐
	Other			
Maternal view	of pain relief post delivery	Very Satisfied ☐	Satisfied ☐	Dissatisfied ☐
Mobilised	since delivery	Y ☐	N ☐	
Passed urine	since delivery	Y ☐	N ☐	
Walked	in labour	Y ☐	N ☐	
Intra-operative discomfort	None ☐ Mild ☐ Moderate ☐	Severe ☐	N/A ☐	

Problems	Royal College of Anaesthetists Severity Score (1 to 5)
☐ **None**	☐
☐ Pruritus	☐
☐ Nausea	☐
☐ Vomiting	☐
☐ Headache	☐
☐ PDPH	☐
☐ Other	☐
Treatment	
☐ Neurological deficit	☐
☐ Motor	☐
☐ Sensory	☐
☐ **Critical incident**	☐
Specify	
☐ ICU ☐ Planned ☐ Unplanned	
☐ HDU ☐ Planned ☐ Unplanned	
☐ Other	

RCA Score

1 Transient abnormality not noticed by patient
2 Transient damage with full recovery
3 Potentially permanent but not disabling damage
4 Potentially disabling damage
5 Death

(Sharpe)EpiduralAnalgesia15273/18109KR

INITIAL DOSE/SPINAL CSE

Mobility Code*			TIME	Drug + Concentration	Vol.	Patient	BP (mins)		Pain Intensity Sco	
B = Bed		U_1 = Standing				Position	5	10	Pre	Post
S = Sitting in chair		U_2 = Walking							None	None
									Mild	Mild
Planned Technique									Moderate	Mode
Top ups	Inf	PCEA							Severe	Sever

Top ups

	MW	Dr	Pt	Spinal						
1st				**Epidural test dose**						
Subsequent										

MAINTENANCE

Time					
Cervical dilatation					
Position of Mother					
Signature					
LA/Opioid	Drug				
	Conc				
	Volume				
Start	Time				
Time	Inf Rate				
Infusion	Vol Inf				
Obs (min) 1=Pre 2=5 3=10 4=15 5=20	1 2 3 4 5	1 2 3 4 5	1 2 3 4 5	1 2
BP				
MHR				
FHR				
Analgesia Score				
Good/Mod/Poor				
Block Height				
Method Te, To, Pi, Ot, #				
Mobility*				
B, S, U_1, U_2				
Infusion Hourly				
Obs Time				
Other				

IMMEDIATE PROBLEMS

None ☐

Failure N ☐ Inadequate ☐ Unilateral ☐ Missed segment ☐ Catheter dislodged ☐
        Y ☐

Intravascular injection ☐ Convulsion ☐ Total spinal ☐ Drug error ☐ Other ☐

bility Code*	TIME of sensory assessment	Sensory Levels				Method		#
		Left		Right		Temperature	Te	
= Bed		U	L	U	L	Touch	To	
= Sitting in chair						Pinprick	Pi	
= Standing						Other	Ot	
= Walking							#	

Reproduced with permission of Miss Obiome Oji

C5
T1
C4
T4
T7
T10
T10
T11
T12
S2/3 L1
L2
L3
L5
S2

Posterior
nerve roots

4	5	1	2	3	4	5	1	2	3	4	5	1	2	3	4	5	1	2	3	4	5

heter N ☐ Catheter N ☐   Special instructions
oved   Y ☐ intact   Y ☐   ....
                                 ....
e   ....
....
                                 ....

Appendix I Recovery chart

TIME INTO RECOVERY _____

LRIMH – Recovery Observation Chart

Every patient requires *continuous* observation by midwife/recovery practitioner for 30 minutes and until all observations are normal and stable. Patients who have received spinal or epidural opioids should remain in recovery for 4 hours after opioid administration to be monitored.

Time after entering recovery	5 min	10 min	20 min	30 min	1 hr	1.5 hr	2 hr	3 hr	4 hr
Time of obs.									
Pulse									
Blood pressure									
SpO2									
Respiratory rate									
Sedation score									
Temperature									
Pain score									
Check wound									
Check PV loss									
Check IV site(s)									
Drain volume									
Urinary cath vol.									
Pt. colour									
Leg power score									

SCORING SYSTEMS

Pulse	if <60 or >100 ⇒ CALL ANAESTHETIST
Blood pressure	if <100 systolic, or >160 systolic or >95 diastolic ⇒ CALL ANAESTHETIST
Pulse oximeter	if <95% ⇒ CALL ANAESTHETIST
Respiratory rate	if <10 ⇒ CALL ANAESTHETIST
Sedation score	0 Awake and Alert 1 Awake but drowsy
	2 Asleep but rousable 3 Unrousable ⇒ CALL ANAESTHETIST
Pain score	none, mild, moderate and severe, if moderate or severe ⇒ CALL ANAESTHETIST
PV loss	if moderate or significant ⇒ CALL ANAESTHETIST/OBSTETRICIAN
Drain volume	if > 200 mls ⇒ CALL ANAESTHETIST/OBSTETRICIAN
Patient colour	if pale or white ⇒ CALL ANAESTHETIST/OBSTETRICIAN
Leg power score	with the women in bed, ask her to draw her heel towards her bottom, one leg at a time
	1 = complete block (unable to move feet or knees)
	2 = almost complete block (able to move feet only)
	3 = partial block (just able to move knees)
	4 = detectable weakness of hip flexion (between 3 & 5)
	5 = no detectable weakness of hip flexion while supine

Index